Every Body's Guide to Everyday Pain

Every Body's Guide to Everyday Pain

"It Never Used to Hurt When I...?!"

YA-LING J. LIOU, D.C.

RETURN TO HEALTH PRESS

SEATTLE, WA

Published by Return to Health Press™, Seattle, WA
Ya-Ling J. Liou, D.C., is a chiropractic physician in Seattle, WA
www.returntohealthpress.com

Notice

The information, techniques and suggestions contained in this book are not intended as a substitute for individual medical care. All matters regarding your health require medical supervision. Consult your health care professional before performing any exercise or taking any dietary supplement referenced in this book. Neither the author, nor the publisher, contributors or editors shall be liable or responsible for any loss, damage or risk arising, directly or indirectly, from the use and application of any of the contents of this book.

The names of all patients have been altered to preserve confidentiality. The details of each clinical anecdote are combinations of excerpts and composites of some of the most common situations.

Cover Design by Bookfly Design
Interior Design by VMC Art & Design, LLC
Photography by Hayden Fidler
Edited by Nancy Wick c/o Enlightened Edits
Research Edits by Sherri Damlo c/o Damlo Does, LLC
Image & Diagram Credits: Diagram 8.3 and 8.5 - Theuplink (2004), *Visceral referred pain areas.* This picture is from Theuplink group (WEBJAUNTE\Michelle); Diagram 9.1 - *Chinese Signs of Five Elements,* © Amiris / Fotolia; Figure 9.1 - *Atlas, or weary man holding up damaged world,* © Richard Miller/Fotolia; Figure 9.2 - *Difficult business task,* © Christos Georghiou/Fotolia

First Edition, 2015
Printed in the United States of America

Library of Congress Control Number: 2015940099
ISBN: 978-09913094-0-5

To each and every one of you who have walked through my office doors and graced my treatment table, this book is for you and because of you. By virtue of your sometimes daring trust in me during some of the most vulnerable times in your life, you've gifted me these insights. These volumes are a collection of all of your shared bodies' wisdom. I am merely the translator.

Namaste.[1]

---

1. One translation of the meaning of the Hindu salutation "Namaste": "*The Divine wisdom in me recognizes and acknowledges the Divine wisdom in you.*"

"The unending paradox is that we do learn through pain."

Madeleine L'Engle

CONTENTS

AUTHOR'S NOTE

FOREWORD

By Joseph Pizzorno, ND

A DIFFICULT CHALLENGE FOR HEALTH CARE professionals is that the majority of our patients will wait until they are seriously suffering before asking for our assistance. Too often this means the underlying causes of their pain have progressed to much more difficult problems. So, how can a person determine whether his or her problem is either self-limiting or can be effectively treated without medical intervention? There is no distinct line, but rather a gray continuum from dysfunction to damage that can be tough to understand for the average person. One solution is to better connect with your body, understand what various kinds and locations of pain mean, recognize what causes the pain, and if the causes will respond to self-care. For those who want to take control of their health, this 3-book series is a marvelous resource.

Pain is nature's way of getting our attention, telling us something is wrong. Our body can be telling us something is damaged and needs a break—for example, when we sprain an ankle and the ankle swells up as a natural splint and hurts so we stop using it—or the body may be telling us that something is not working right, like when we get severe leg pain while walking when the arteries to the legs are so blocked there is not enough blood supply for our muscles to work properly. Another example is the buildup of toxins in the body when we have a hangover after consuming too much alcohol. All of these signs are important, and each has a different cause and each requires a different intervention.

Conventional medicine has become extremely good at developing drugs, and even surgical procedures, to turn off these important messages. The many drugs, especially those called nonsteroidal anti-inflammatory drugs (NSAIDs), are readily available as prescriptions and over-the-counter formulations. For short-term use, they can provide effective relief. However, the larger challenge is that simply turning off the body's messages is not a great strategy for health.

It is worth underscoring that occasional and limited use of NSAIDs is typically not problematic, but it cannot be emphasized enough that the long-term use of NSAIDs to *ignore* the body's messages can lead to serious—and sometimes permanent—damage. Therefore, it's important to learn from the information contained in *Every Body's Guide to Everyday Pain*, which is an excellent resource to help you recognize and address those underlying causes of pain, rather than simply taking drugs to mask the pain signals your body is trying to communicate to you.

PREFACE

THE INTENTION AND DRIVE TO CREATE this three-book series came simply from a desire to fill a need that I saw in my own practice. I was wishing for a comprehensive patient guide that I could send home with people because I often found myself wanting more time but having to leave patients with what I considered to be only a morsel of the big picture about how to manage the pain, get better and learn to avoid recurring episodes.

I've seen many good books about back pain, but the information is frequently offered in a way that strikes me as difficult to use from the practical point of view of someone who is in significant discomfort and needs answers right away. Before any resolution is possible, we need to be able to wrap our minds around the reasons for our everyday pain. Once we grasp firstly that our pain makes sense and secondly that we'll be okay, then we can better conceptualize what to do right this minute in order to manage the situation, avoid making it worse and, finally, learn how to keep from having the whole experience all over again. What you'll find in *Volume One—Put Out the Fire* is the first step in this progression, including some basic accessible information in order to quickly and effectively diffuse the stress of the situation and set the stage for success.

It was my goal to create the kind of trouble-shooting guide for everyday pain that would serve to offer help for use during early stages of healing. I also find it important to include an honest and well-rounded snapshot of *all* contributing factors to pain. It's not *just* your posture. It's not the suboptimal eating and sleeping habits *alone*. It's not *only* that you're stressed or depressed. It's every single one of these things to varying degrees for each of us at alternating times in our lives. While this may seem like an overwhelming idea, it's actually completely within your reach to understand and transform.

When I am guiding my patients along the path back to health and out of pain, I want them to become aware of not just the mechanical factors at play but also the biochemical and emotional aspects that are often the things that need attention in order to achieve complete and lasting resolution. My work as a chiropractor has little lasting impact if the issues of biochemistry and life coping skills are ignored. Imbalance in any one of these three areas (mechanics, biochemistry and emotions) can significantly contribute to pain and dysfunction, which means that, in order to influence successful recovery, these same factors must be equally addressed through all stages of injury and healing.

Any of the popular "quick fixes" for health and wellness that sound catchy, trendy and easy all work for short periods of time because there is *some* truth in all of them, but it's never long before another imbalance arises and calls for attention. Until we stop allowing ourselves to be seduced by the distracting notion of a "quick fix" and start instead thinking about the big picture, we will continue to experience episodes of pain and the quest for balanced health will continue to be a frustrating game of hit or miss.

There is no reason in my mind that we shouldn't have perfectly good command of the workings of our own body, but, unfortunately, information about health is often presented in a way that perpetuates an illusion of scientific mysticism— something to be handed down only by the "experts." Unfortunately, much of this "expert" advice, while presenting helpful information, also often perpetuates some commonly held beliefs about posture and movement that are incorrect, easily misinterpreted or can very possibly make things worse. Professional input is invaluable but only to the extent that it helps you realize that with the *right* guidance, in the end, you are actually your own best expert. This book is designed to serve as just such a resource—a supplement, an educational reference and support for the times when professional help might not be immediately available during the inevitable, unexpected episodes of everyday pain.

INTRODUCTION

The Three Big Questions

ARE YOU SOMEONE WHO'S DONE ROUNDS with massage thera-pists, chiropractors, physical therapists, acupuncturists, orthopedists or perhaps even physiatrists (the newer hybridized medical physicians who straddle the world of orthopedics, neurology and physical rehabilitation)? Have you been told there's nothing wrong with you, that no one seems to have a really clear explanation of why you're having pain, and yet a couple times a year or more you just wake up with it? Do you feel like you're not doing anything out of the ordinary that would justify the pain you deal with? Maybe you get up off the couch one day and, suddenly, there it is again! Or is it while simply sitting still at your computer, you find yourself hit with that familiar burning ache or stabbing pinch? If you are willing to face the possibility that it's *not* just old age and that there *is* an easier, more pain-free, day-to-day exis-tence out there for you, then you should dive head first into this book.

On the other hand, if you are still holding out hope for a quick fix, this is probably not the book for you because you won't find that here. In the modern world, a multitude of methods, supplements, dietary modifications, exercises, and ways of life exist that are touted by so-called experts as the great panacea to what ails any and all of us. Unfortunately, the reality is that no single one of these so-called cures works for all people at all times, nor for all purposes.

What *does* work 100% of the time, however, is better understanding our body—its limitations and potentials. Only then can we, with confidence and calm, navigate the ups and downs of life with this physical form of ours as it takes us from childhood through old age. To do so with as much ease of body *and* mind as possible is, in my opinion, the best we can strive for. Just a little bit of guidance combined with our own inquisitiveness can help each of us learn to be our own expert when it comes to everyday aches and pains. What every one of us needs first is to be shown how to tap into what we already instinctively know. We need to return to our body's innate common sense. We all deserve to find ways to return to health, and by picking up this book you've started down the right path. Get ready to think critically and befriend your body.

As you read, it's important to keep in mind that the kind of pain I'm talking about in this book is the "everyday" variety—a fairly average array of physical aches and pains. It is assumed that blood tests, internal exams, magnetic resonance imaging and X-rays have ruled out serious underlying causes. If you have any doubt about your own pain, make sure to seek help sooner rather than later. You should *not* consider this book a substitute for medical help. It is intended only to be a supplement that will help you get the most out of bodywork or any other professional guidance you choose to pursue. There is never any good substitute for a fresh and professional perspective on whatever ails us.

I have spent more than 20 years as a chiropractor helping my patients through a wide array of painful situations. Throughout the years what I've found is that, while there is simply no single "right" answer for all of us, there are some common principles that can shed a good amount of light on these following three questions: (1) "Why does it hurt?"; (2) "How do I make it stop?"; and (3) "How do I keep it from happening again?" The answers to each of these questions come from an understanding of some of the universal mechanical and chemical challenges that the human body is exposed to on a day-to-day basis. As it turns out, our body's responses to these challenges are actually completely predictable. What is *not* so predictable is the variable threshold at which each of us hits our "breaking point," which is what leads us to the experience of pain—not to mention the many individual ways in which pain is felt and expressed.

A large part of what I love about my work is exactly this unique variability of each person's response to treatment. This constant variability is part of what keeps me engaged and thinking on my feet. Despite the wide variation of individuals, cases and outcomes, over the years it's become clear to me that there are numerous universal triggers of everyday pain and it's simply this *variable tolerance* of ours for imperfect circumstances that can make it seem confusing.

These universal triggers of everyday pain fall into one of three categories: mechanical, chemical or emotional. All three of these stressors can influence each other as well. Everyday pain triggers often stay just under the radar, thanks to the body's adaptive capabilities. When we finally do feel pain, it can seem like it's coming from "out of the blue" because generally it's the result of having reached our limit of adaptive capability, just like a bucket brimming with water can suddenly overflow with one last drop. Part of the detective work that I do in my office with patients, aside from finding and fixing restricted joints, involves tracing the pain back to a key trigger for that particular individual's situation. Figuring out what the primary trigger might have been gives him or her the best chance to rehabilitate properly from that specific mechanism of strain, but it also helps that person avoid undoing all of my hard work as soon as he or she returns to day-to-day habits.

It's my job to help restore mechanical function to areas of the body that have been trying to adapt to some of these triggers by becoming restricted or locked up. My work starts with the spine, and the initial intent is to address mechanics, but it's hard to deny the interconnectedness of all other body systems as they display their own response to those changes made at the spine. The spine is essentially a stack of bones connected by joint capsules, disk cushions and ligaments. These capsules, disks and ligaments lie directly next to and rub up against muscle tendons (where they attach to bones) and muscle bellies (the meaty, fleshy parts).

All of these structures—bones to muscles and everything in between—are richly awash in blood, nerve cells and lymph vessels that react, then relay and receive information to and from the brain, and, in turn, to and from the rest of the body, including our vital organs. This is not unlike how one drop of water into a pond creates ripples far from where that drop lands. A single helpful maneuver to the spine, for example, can cause a cascade of effects among all of the interrelated structures and systems of the body and brain. Unfortunately, this is also true of any single negative or stressful event, big or small, anywhere in the body.

Witnessing this clinical interconnectedness in daily practice gives me the broad perspective from which this book was created and inspires me to share my insights. I am indebted to my patients who've trusted me time and again to help them troubleshoot their pain and guide them to find their way out of it. My work with patients continues to confirm for me that it's important to remember the neurobiochemical influences that can profoundly change the mechanical aspect of function or dysfunction when treating pain. Neurobiochemistry affects all tissues and organs of the body. Despite how intimidating that word "neurobiochemical" may sound to some, it boils down to some very common sense ideas that you'll see more of in the very first chapter.

Read on. Enjoy the adventure into the workings of your body and see where it takes you.

Section I:

Why Does it Hurt?

CHAPTER 1

Inflammation: Your Body on Fire

THE EASIEST ANSWER TO THE QUESTION of why it hurts is that pain is the result of inflammation. There are chemicals that build up in our tissues during an inflammatory response along with swelling, and it's these chemicals that are responsible for causing pain and irritation. It's really as plain as that. You might be thinking, "No, no, no, *my* pain is all about my tight muscles." Well, guess what? You won't find the one (muscle pain and tightness) without some degree of the other (inflammation). A *tight* muscle group can exist for quite some time without hurting. The *pain* or sensation of a tight muscle is what we feel when inflammation over-whelms the region.

So, if inflammation is what really lies at the heart of all pain in one form or another,

> "Pain is the result of inflammation"

what exactly is it? Simply put: inflammation is a sudden increase in blood flow. Generally we consider increased blood flow to be a good thing. Blood does nourish all the tissues in the body by delivering nutrients and oxygen everywhere. Unfortunately, just a little more than usual of this good thing can make everything feel quite wrong. There are many different scenarios in which inflammation is at play in unexpected and subtle ways.

We can easily see that inflammation is at play with something as obvious as a twisted ankle. If you've ever had an ankle sprain you'll remember there was redness, a feeling of heat and a good amount of noticeable puffiness that makes it hard to keep a snug shoe on for too long after the sprain occurs. But the classic signs of redness, heat and swelling aren't always this obvious with inflammation; many cases of pain that come with sensations of muscle tightness and aching are actually manifestations of inflammation as well. Whether or not we can see the clear changes, the process is exactly the same no matter where in the body or in what group of tissues it's occurring.

Think of inflammation as your body on fire. Sometimes a white hot coal doesn't look hot at all until you poke it and sparks fly.

The tissues of the body from deepest to most superficial include: bones, joint capsules, ligaments, muscles, fascia and skin (Figure 1.1).

Irritation to any of these will result in some degree of inflammation. When the surface of the skin is inflamed from a scrape, for example, we can clearly see it and feel it: redness, heat and swelling. When the joints, ligaments and muscles are irritated and inflamed, the exact same process is going on, but on the inside—out of plain view.

Think about what happens when there is repeated irritation to any one portion of the skin—for example, from wearing an ill-fitting shoe. First, blisters may form on numerous occasions. Then, if irritation continues, the body learns and will adapt. Adaptation is a way of maintaining a semblance of function while under stress. In the case of repeatedly irritated skin over a long period of time, we may eventually develop a callus. A callus is a thicker, protective, less flexible layer of tissue in an area of chronic irritation. The *exact same thing* can happen on the *inside* of the body. There are various forms of internal, musculoskeletal equivalents of a skin callus, and these are what we sometimes refer to as adhesions, knots, or even bone spurs. They also are the result of exposure to repeated and prolonged stress—often involving friction of some sort.

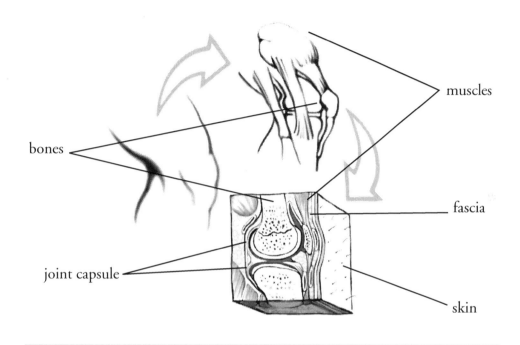

FIGURE 1.1 TISSUES OF THE BODY: Notice how intimately all the tissues of the body relate to each other. From superficial to deep: skin, fascia, muscles, more fascia, joint capsules then bone.

If we know that something like repeated rubbing from the pressure of a shoe is a plainly recognizable source of irritation for the skin of our feet, then we can choose to avoid wearing that shoe. What we should ask ourselves now is: "What sorts of things are considered irritating to bones, joints, ligaments and muscles that may result in the forming of similarly adaptive responses like adhesions (what we think of as muscle knots) or bone spurs?" We'll look more closely at this once we gain a better understanding of what inflammation really is so that we know what we're dealing with. Once we become more familiar with the kinds of possible tissue irritants, we have a better chance of resolving the associated pain or avoiding them and the pain altogether.

Inflammation: Your Body on Fire

Inflammation is essentially your body or body part or group of tissues on fire. We know that fire can be very destructive if left unchecked and it can also be a very efficient way to do away with waste. The fire of inflammation behaves in much the same way. Injury or strain to any tissue of the body results in a break-down of that particular tissue and causes the production of a larger-than-usual amount of cellular waste. Cellular waste is being produced all the time as part of the natural process of living and breathing, but it's the sudden and larger-than-usual amount of waste after injury that can only be disposed of effectively by setting it on fire.

If left to accumulate, the build-up of cellular waste can cause further stress on the already injured area and possibly neighboring tissues as well. So setting it on fire is the right thing to do (inflammation is good); unfortunately, the resulting fire of inflammation can itself become very uncomfortable. Most cases of inflammation are self-limiting and simply part and parcel of a healthy repair process, but sometimes when conditions are just so, the fire of inflammation can continue out of control. It may start simmering just under the surface—ready to flare up unexpectedly at any time, or it can stay flared up long past its usefulness following injury if we don't tend to the needs of an injured or stressed part of the body.

When any part of the body is under stress, the temperature gets turned up, so to speak. Whether or not this stress turns into an inflammatory fire depends on a number of factors. If you put yourself on a treadmill, for example, your body will experience a type of treadmill-induced stress. How do you know? You get warm, maybe flushed, and you produce sweat. Heat, redness and swelling—only imagine that the swelling in this example is escaping through your pores in the form of sweat. These are your signs of treadmill stress. If the treadmill is set to a high speed you're bound to feel very warm and get red in the face and probably soak through your shirt in no time. Those signs of stress will be very dramatic. Similarly, a sudden and severe stress anywhere in the body will result in an obvious display of inflammation like that of a sprained ankle (Figure 1.2A).

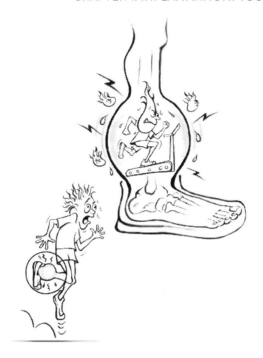

FIGURE 1.2A ACUTE INFLAMMATION—SUDDEN INJURY: The acute inflammation of sudden injury leads to swelling, heat and redness that we can easily see.

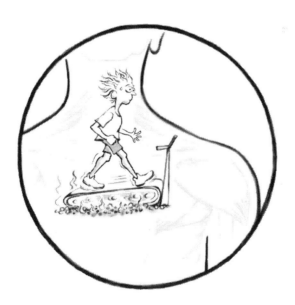

FIGURE 1.2B LOW-GRADE SIMMERING INFLAMMATION: The low-grade simmering inflammation of everyday pain can lurk undetected for weeks, months or even years.

> "Adaptation is a way of maintaining a semblance of function while under stress."

If you get on a treadmill set to a leisurely speed, it will take you a long time to notice those signs of stress and they may be very mild: A little bit of color in the face, eventually you get warm enough to peel off a layer of clothing and maybe your forehead beads up a bit …but probably not before an hour or so goes by. Similarly, a minor tissue strain will result in signs of stress that the body can handle and keep under control for a long time before we really notice anything at all (Figure 1.2B).

This—the situation in Figure 1.2B—is the kind of situation I see in my office all the time. I can't tell you how many times I hear, "I just woke up with it," especially in the case of neck and shoulder pain. Or I'll hear, "I was just sitting comfortably, relaxing but then when I got up," which is very common with the onset of the everyday variety of lower back pain. Everyday pain very often seems to hit out of the blue, without any dramatic injury, and this can be some of the most perplexing pain there is. Consider the stories of three patients of mine:

When Everyday Pain Hits Out of the Blue

Ed the carpenter suffers an unexpected "danger" in his bedtime routine:

ED is a 42-year-old male patient who has seen me fairly infrequently, but when he has, it's been for chronic, recurrent mid-back pain and tightness. He works as a carpenter and enjoys his craft. He recently returned for treatment, but for pain in the lower back this time. He says there wasn't anything sudden or obvious that led to this pain. Driving home from work he noticed a little bit of tightness and he felt stiff getting out of the car. That evening he played one of his 4-year-old son's favorite games, holding him on his arms outstretched over the bed. Ed pretends he is a frying pan and his son likes to imagine that he is a burger in the frying pan about to be flipped, and then he does get flipped right onto the bed in fits of squealing laughter. Pretty darn sweet.

All of that horsing around (surprisingly and horrifyingly to the chiropractor in me) usually goes off with no injuries to either party as it did again that night. Who can resist this kind of gleeful play with their child at the end of a dull workday? The rest of the evening goes well and after dinner there is some time spent unwinding on the couch. Getting up from the couch an hour later, Ed notices that same stiffness in the lower back that he felt in the car on the way home. Thinking nothing of it, he makes his way to bed, stopping in the bathroom to brush his teeth.

Standing at the bathroom sink, he's barely had a chance to reach for the toothpaste when he feels a sharp, blinding pain in his lower back and shooting into the buttock. It took his breath away for a split second and he had to grab onto the sink to keep from buckling at the knees. For someone who uses his body vigorously on a daily basis, feeling so severely injured by such a ridiculously, non-athletic event doesn't make any sense at all. He puts himself to bed thinking this pain is nonsense and maybe it'll just go away after a good night's rest...

Charlene, the dancer and yoga teacher caught unaware
doing nothing more than casually walking:

CHARLENE is a 32-year-old female patient of mine who is a modern dancer and a yoga instructor. She currently does more teaching and choreography than dancing. The reason Charlene finds herself in my office on this particular occasion is because of a sharp pain in the mid-back that seems to stab right through to the chest, taking her breath away. All she was doing when it struck was walking from her car into a store. This is a pain Charlene has never experienced in all of her years of pushing her body to various physical limits, and here it is, so debilitating and yet with seemingly no perceivable trauma leading up to it…

Billie the office worker injured while "resting":

BILLIE is a 52-year-old woman in administrative management and has no interest in pushing her body or testing her physical limits. Even if that sort of thing interested her, she has absolutely no time these days. When she has a free moment the only thing she wants to do is sleep or collapse and unwind from her day. By looking at her, you would not think she is out of shape, but Billie tells me she is just completely wrung out at the end of each day and longs for the time when it seemed like she had so much more energy—she felt so much healthier back then. Other than an increase in age and a decline in her work satisfaction, not much else has changed. She's never been active but has always had a strong body with no problems other than some knee pain that has slowly been getting worse. Her daily life consists of hours at a desk with a computer and a phone.

Billie had been meaning to come and see me for a few months about a set of symptoms she wasn't even sure was anything I could help her with. Well, before she even had a chance to be seen for that problem, she found herself going to bed one night after a long day with nothing out of the ordinary standing out, yet waking in the morning feeling as if she had turned into Quasimodo (in her words). Her neck was completely frozen up and hurting as never before. She could barely pick her head up off of the pillow and it brought tears to her eyes when she finally did—only with the help of her own hands. Billie is not an athlete, she did nothing out of her ordinary routine and, yet, suffered what another patient of mine coined a "sleeping injury." Sometimes the most perplexing pain happens to us while we're lying in bed at night, trying recharge our batteries. I see it time and again...

When everyday pain suddenly hits us, what's happened is that part of the tissue repair system has gotten overwhelmed and has backed up. After quietly accumulating from days, weeks or months of low-grade repetitive strain, those pain-causing byproducts of stress can unexpectedly spill over like a bucket that has been brimming for quite some time and then takes just one last drop too many. What our everyday pain buckets are brimming with is caustic, irritating but perfectly natural cellular waste. Often the final drop in the bucket is nothing more than a movement or position that we would normally consider to be completely non-traumatic and maybe even routine—like our favorite sleeping position, sitting on the couch or reaching for the toothpaste. The bucket overflows and we suddenly find ourselves in an alarming amount of pain with little or no warning. It often does not take much to disrupt what has been up to that point a delicate balance about which we were previously completely oblivious—thanks to the body's ability to adapt (Figures 1.3A and 1.3B).

It's easy to get angry and frustrated when pain comes out of nowhere like this, especially if we have no way of understanding *what* happened or why. With a little more information we don't have to feel so helpless. So, let's dig in, and figure it out once and for all!

Here's how the everyday pain bucket fills up: Stressed tissue (muscles, tendons, ligaments, joints and all the spaces, cells and membranes in between) produces a molecular "sweat" of sorts—just like you would on a treadmill. These cellular signs of stress trigger a relief-and-repair response via the circulatory system, which acts as the body's transport system. This circulatory transport system is designed to get nutrients and waste shuttled around the body to the appropriate locations. Networks of blood vessels will open up or "dilate" around the stressed or injured area—just like streets will clear out (or are supposed to) when emergency vehicles are on their way to the scene of an injury. Normally, when tissue stress is occurring at a low level and all systems are working optimally, the bucket gets emptied almost as quickly as it gets filled.

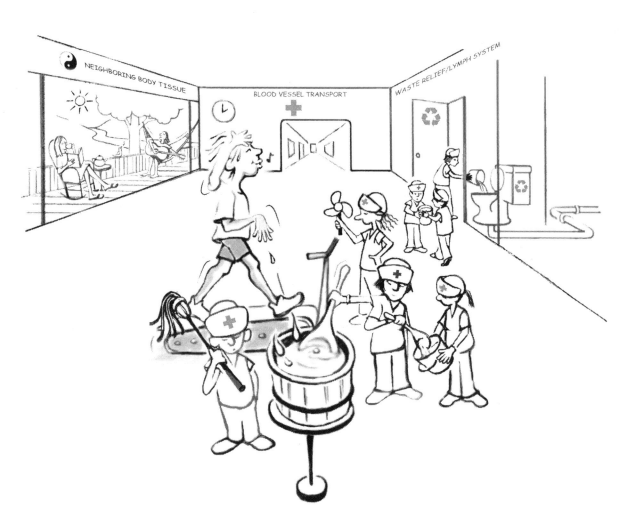

FIGURE 1.3A STRESS OF NORMAL DAILY ACTIVITIES WITH NO PAIN:
The stress of normal daily activities produces waste just like the sweat you see here gathering in the bucket. But here its production rate is well within the tissue clean-up crew's capacity. It's just an ordinary day of cell and tissue metabolism.

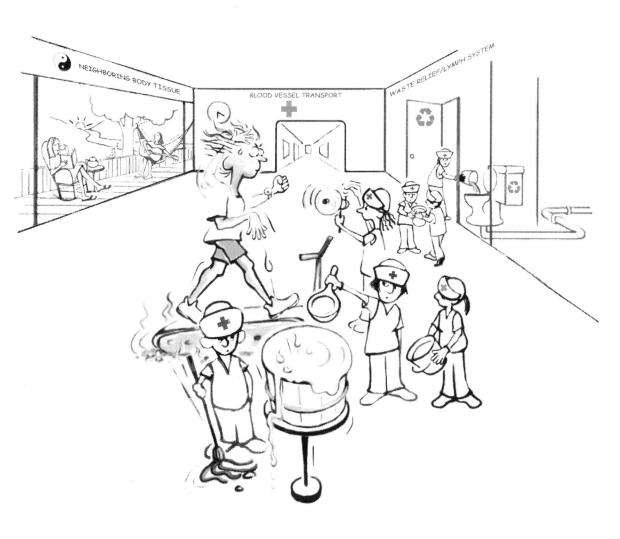

**FIGURE 1.3B ACCUMULATION OF THE PRECURSORS TO INFLAM-
MATION:** Add some low-grade additional stressors to the
stress of normal daily activities and you start to see the waste
accumulation nearing the clean-up crew's maximum capacity.
Still no pain *but* the bucket is brimming, and simmering coals
(precursors to inflammation) begin to gather and lurk.

> "Most cases of inflammation are self limiting and simply part and parcel of a healthy repair process"

In the case of overwhelming inflammation that we see with pain, getting aid vehicles (our cellular relief-and-repair response) to the scene is rarely a problem for the body, but getting them *out* of there at the same rate of speed to make room for more relief workers or clean-up crew, is not so easy. The redness, heat and swelling of crisis-level inflammation is what happens when these "aid vehicles" and all the other cellular "traffic" in the area gets backed up. This traffic jam process is the same for sudden injury as well as for what's referred to as an "insidious" onset—situations with no clear cause. The bigger and more concentrated the traffic jam, the more pain there will be. First there is the mechanical pressure from the circulatory fluids (blood and lymph) pressing up against pain-sensitive neighboring structures. The actual pressure of that sort of crowding in the tissues causes pain and stress of its own.

As if this weren't uncomfortable enough, the chemical build-up of inflammatory byproducts (the smoke and flames of the fire) cause *molecular* irritation to the nerve endings in the area. The molecular "sweat" of stressed tissue along with the resultant figurative ash and fumes of this inflammation fire is like a corrosive substance that the emergency personnel are trying to shuttle out of the area. But when the size of the back-up exceeds the capacity of our relief-and-repair aid personnel, the area becomes overwhelmed, thus allowing the irritating byproducts to accumulate and fester (Figures 1.4A and 1.4B).

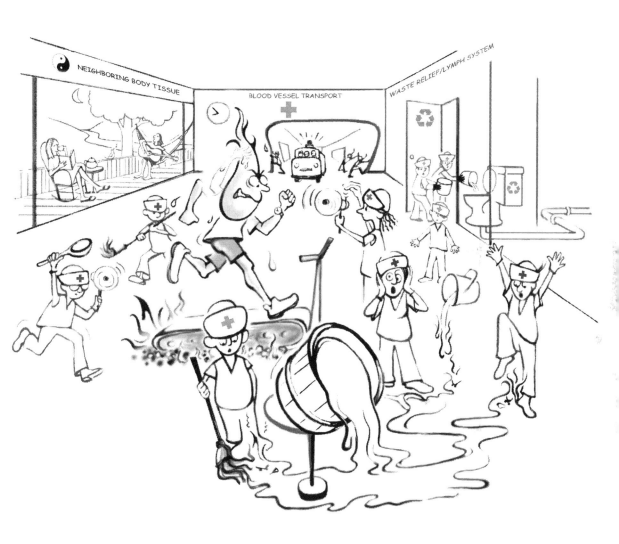

FIGURE 1.4A INFLAMMATION SIMMERING JUST BELOW THE SURFACE: When the stress of normal daily activities is paired with low-grade additional inflammatory conditions over time, it takes no more than a single additional drop into the waste bucket to cause an overflow and trigger our body's emergency response...and so begins the *pain* of inflammation.

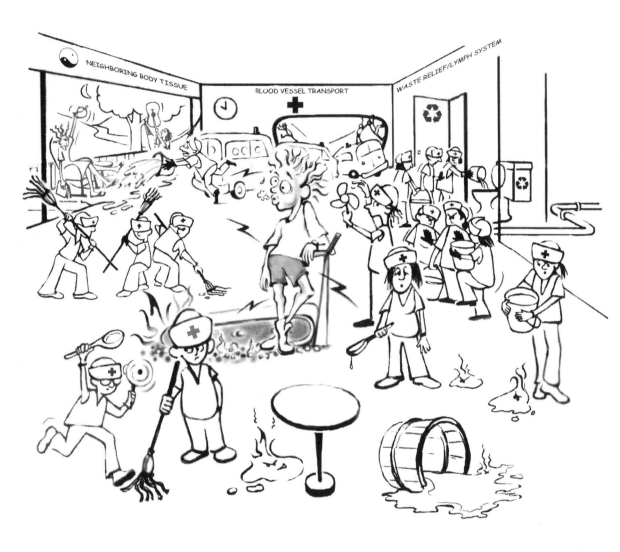

FIGURE 1.4B FULL-BLOWN INFLAMMATION: The source of stress is gone but the tissues are now damaged. Repair has been initiated but there is overcrowding of tired clean-up molecules and now neighboring body tissues might begin suffering some of the inflammation overload as well. The most talked about part of pain is the fallout from precisely this cellular "traffic jam" mayhem.

The painful back-up and build-up of injured tissue waste, in combination with noxious inflammatory byproducts, *can* be controlled. All we need to do is to manage the three different components of the relief-and-repair traffic jam to keep clean-up efforts flowing:

1. You've got to first **stop the stress signal** responsible for summoning all of the "aid vehicles" with clean-up crew on board. If it's the treadmill, as in my analogy, then get off the treadmill! Stopping the stress signal means you have to stop doing the things that cause the hurt. Sounds easy, but sometimes the things that cause the pain aren't obvious to us.

2. Next, you can work on **relieving the "traffic" congestion** from all of those aid vehicles already on the scene, not to mention the mess left by the stress-damaged tissue. Open up circulatory pathways around the injury (increase hallway size). Clear the immediate area around the treadmill (the tissue *next to* the stressed tissue) so that the first-aid workers and clean-up crew can come take care of the mess (put out the rest of the fire, sweep up the ashes and blow out the smoke).

3. Finally, you've got to **keep it up!** Keep things moving/flowing (encourage aid workers to keep working until the fire is completely out). How do you help the clean-up crew keep cleaning? You take care of them. Let them eat and rest. Bring in replacements. Make sure lines of communication stay open so that they don't stop work prematurely. Hopefully you've nurtured a good relationship with the place that supplies the aid vehicles and workers so that when you need their help they'll show up in good shape. Taking care of your mechanical, chemical and emotional health is what determines the quality of your body's response to stress.

Control the jam and you control the pain. Specific aspects of inflammatory byproduct "traffic jam" control through movement, nutrient intake and attention to your emotions will be examined with increasing detail in Section II: How Do I Make it Stop?

Triggers of Inflammation

So, what *are* these situations that can cause the tissues of the body to send inflammation-causing stress signals in the first place? And why does this sudden painful back-up of inflammation happen? We can't control factors that we don't understand, so let's take a look. In many cases the answers may be simpler than we imagine—but only if we pay attention to them right away. People who have learned to put up with pain on a daily basis teach their body and nervous system to ignore important warning signs. When things are finally "bad enough" to feel attention is warranted, the situation can be so convoluted and veiled in protective or compensatory layers that it becomes a very long road back to being pain free. The pain of inflammation even just slightly out of control is the body's primary way to communicate to us about anything it perceives to be an irritant—a burden. Sometimes the irritant is fairly obvious, like a sports injury, but most of the time our everyday pain is from something much more subtle and deceptively familiar.

It's not hard to see that inflammation is one of the body's main adaptive responses to stress and injury. What you might find surprising, though, is the wide variety of situations that are actually considered by the brain to be stressful or injurious. Many of them don't involve anything sudden or very obvious at all. Many types of stress and strain are the result of prolonged imbalance. There can be either *mechanical* imbalance or *chemical* imbalance. How and to what degree these two types of imbalances affect us sometimes has to do with a third type of imbalance: emotional. Just as emotions are real physical and chemical experiences, our mechanical and chemical dynamics profoundly influence our emotions. We will take a closer look at all of these with increasing detail throughout all three volumes of this book series.

Our ongoing struggle to physically balance different parts of our body while moving upright against gravity provides many opportunities for *mechanical* stress, while a dizzying combination of genetics, toxin or allergen load and nutrient intake dictate how *chemically* vulnerable our tissues are to physiological stress or imbalance. So, on a daily basis, we're either doing our darnedest to balance the structural load of various body parts (both when they are in motion and when they are still) against the forces of gravity, or we're navigating a delicate dance between what boils down to "garbage in vs. garbage out." Since inflammation or, using the analogy, a body "on fire" is basically a body doing its best to repair itself, we know the intention is good; the combustion of fire *is* after all very helpful at breaking down waste, and waste is exactly what is produced by any stressed and injured tissue.

"Inflammation is one of the body's main adaptive responses to stress and injury."

While tissue stressors or irritants are fairly universal and predictable, individual tolerance varies widely from person to person. There are countless things that we do or subject ourselves to in daily life that are potential irritants to our muscles and joints or organ systems, but because each body has such a wildly differing composition of mechanical and chemical resilience, not everyone responds or reacts in the same way to the same degree of irritation.

Think of the treadmill example again for a minute. Five different people walking at the same speed for the same amount of time will show five individual displays of treadmill stress at different moments. These differences will depend on their fitness level, energy level, when and what they last ate or drank, as well as individual performance potential based on genetics—just to mention a few variables. Whether or not we see the effects right away, in this example the treadmill is the indisputable and universal source of stress. We see that there is high variability in how the effects of this stress are manifested and experienced by the person subjected to them. But accepting the fact that being on the treadmill is a universal source of stress, we can better see that, first of all, whatever the response to it, it is not unreasonable; secondly, it gives us a starting point for figuring out what needs to change.

Mechanical stressors (in this example, it's movement against gravity) can and do often coexist with chemical stressors (tissue waste, along with the "smoke" and "flames" of the clean-up effort). Sometimes it's the chemical overload and other times it's one mechanical irritation too many that tips the scale, pushing us to a painful state. Similarly, either one of those irritants (chemistry or mechanics) can be responsible for low-grade simmering inflammation that goes undetected for years. Very often, by the time we feel pain, both mechanics and chemistry are at play to some degree. As alluded to earlier, in some cases we might find that both are actually strongly influenced by lesser acknowledged but sometimes extremely pertinent and deeply ingrained emotional factors as well. We will continue to take a closer look at all three of these sources of stress and causes of pain—mechanics, chemistry and emotions—as they relate to each other.

CHAPTER 2

Mechanical Triggers

TISSUES OF THE BODY CAN EXPERIENCE mechanical injury when *structural* integrity is threatened. Some examples of mechanical stress or mechanical triggers of inflammation include:

- Compression (compressive forces)
- Lengthening, i.e., any positioning of body parts at some distance from our individual center of gravity (tensile force)
- Shearing forces that result from combining compression and tension

> "The spine experiences and negotiates the compressive force of gravity all day long."

Compression

Compressive forces can come from gravity or from a crushing type of injury (Figure 2.1).

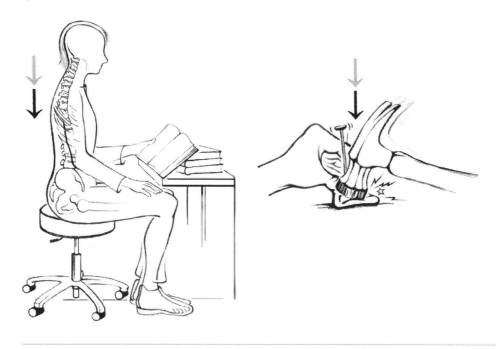

FIGURE 2.1 COMPRESSION—A MECHANICAL STRESS: Compression is a mechanical stress that can trigger pain. The spine experiences and negotiates the compressive force of gravity all day long. Gravity is a significant compressive force all on its own, but, combine that with a blow or a fall, and we have a reasonable mechanical trigger for pain.

Lengthening

Tensile forces from a lengthening stress can come from active stretching, sustained postural quirks and any number of routine tasks if they occur in an unbalanced way that may be perceived by the brain as a threat to our postural balance (Figure 2.2).

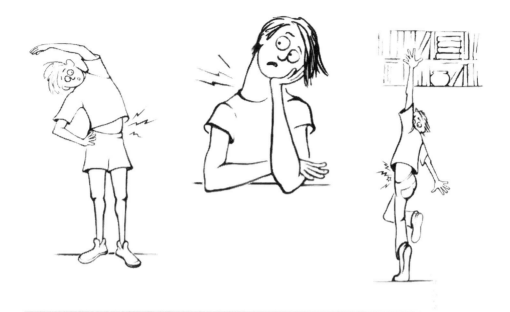

FIGURE 2.2 LENGTHENING—A MECHANICAL STRESS: Lengthening is another mechanical stress that can trigger pain. Moving two attached objects away from each other will always stress the connection between them. Our tissue elasticity is what allows us to experience some lengthening without pain, but the stress caused by lengthening exists whether or not we feel it.

Shearing

Shearing is a type of injury seen most commonly at the level of our spinal disks. Anyone who's ever had a disk injury knows that the most perfect recipe for disaster is twisting and bending at the same time—even without picking up anything heavy. The cushioning and the joint capsules that connect our spinal bones can become inflamed to varying degrees if they undergo shearing stress. Repeated shearing irritation at the disks can lead to bulges or herniations, but most back pain occurs as an early warning system *before* there is real damage to the disks (Figure 2.3). The effect of shearing forces can also be seen with plant-and-pivot knee injuries to the meniscus.

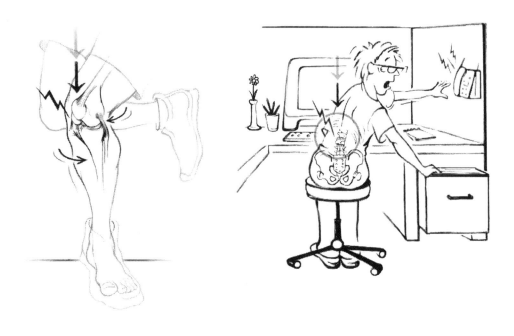

FIGURE 2.3 SHEARING—A MECHANICAL STRESS: Shearing is a mechanical stress that results from the combination of compression and lengthening. Often the lengthening happening with shearing forces is in the form of twisting, and this twisting happens around our Y axis rather than around the X axis that we saw with common examples of lengthening. (Imagine the Y axis line extending from your head to your feet and the X axis extending from right to left.)

Everyone's brain holds something of a blueprint that outlines parameters of acceptable physiological standards for survival. For example, there are subconscious settings in the brain that keep the lungs breathing and keep the heart beating when we sleep—so even when we surrender conscious control the brain makes sure we meet these standards for survival. Part of that blueprint also includes information about where the body can physically be in space with the least amount of muscular effort and work. Because of the interdependence between the organ systems of the body and the structure that houses them, the physical placement of the body can be theoretically equally important to survival by ensuring the most optimal environment for these life-sustaining systems to do their job (Figure 2.4).

This mechanical "optimal" neutral zone is unique to each individual physique (shape and size) and any movements or positions that occur outside of, or deviate from, our individual optimal zone quickly trigger a protective and stabilizing reaction by the central nervous system. The central nervous system is, in effect, focused twenty-four hours a day, seven days a week, on preventing compromised organ function based on the information in our individual blueprints. This established neutral zone is our reference point for how best to avoid falling over or collapsing in different directions against gravity, thereby also naturally protecting our disks, bones, ligaments and tendons from injury—another important survival reflex.

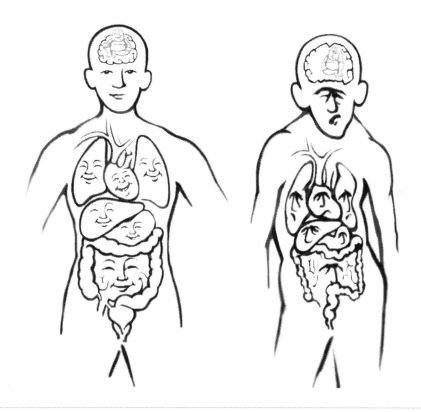

FIGURE 2.4 WELL-HOUSED INTERNAL ORGANS VS. COMPROMISED INTERNAL ORGANS DUE TO POSTURE: On the left-hand side we see an example of optimal body posture providing the correct amount of space for optimal organ functioning. On the right-hand side we see what happens with a collapse in posture and in extreme situations this can compromise organ functioning.

This righting mechanism is a fairly brilliant adaptive feature that allows us to overcome a wide host of situations that the body may or may not be ideally equipped for. If, for example, part of us leans to the left, then the muscles on the right side of the body engage in order to control the movement. Assuming we are strong and muscularly well balanced, once we complete a task requiring us to lean to the left, those same muscles on the right side that just kept us from falling over in the direction we were leaning are supposed to disengage as we return to neutral. With that return to neutral, balance is restored and life carries on until next time.

However, with the demands of modern living, our one-sided leaning tasks can go on for hours and often exceed the natural capacity of those stabilizing muscles on the opposite side (Figure 2.5). But despite the excessive demand, rather than giving out on us, the body recruits neighboring muscles to lend a helping hand (Figure 2.6).

If we exhaust even the help of those backup muscles, *then* we're left with no other choice but to begin forming adhesions. Bands of connective tissue in and around muscles get stuck together and end up exerting a shrink-wrapping effect on all the tissues in the immediate area. This shrink-wrapping adhesion actually gives us exactly what we need—extra *tensile* strength—when we find ourselves short on sufficient muscular endurance[2] for the job at hand, which in many cases is something simple, like getting engrossed in a project at the computer with our head and shoulders craned forward or to one side.

Unfortunately, the stickiness of adhesions causes friction with neighboring tissue, and friction results in irritation and, inevitably, inflammation. This shrink-wrapping effect also—just as it sounds—partially but effectively asphyxiates the tissues in the process, and, in exchange for this increased stability, we develop rigidity and lose the ability to take up normal blood flow with oxygen and nutrients. In the absence of nutrients delivered by way of free blood circulation, the muscles and surrounding soft tissues are slowly forced to transform from soft, juicy and pliable to rigid, inflexible and sinewy (Figure 2.7).

---

2. The muscular endurance needed to sustain the inherently stressful mechanical scenarios of modern living can be insufficient even in the most athletic and physically fit individual. It is reasonable to find just as many stress points and adhesions in a muscularly, well-developed body as it is in a couch potato. The difference that matters between these two body types is the rate of recovery. A fit individual will without a doubt recover more quickly from any injury than an inactive person.

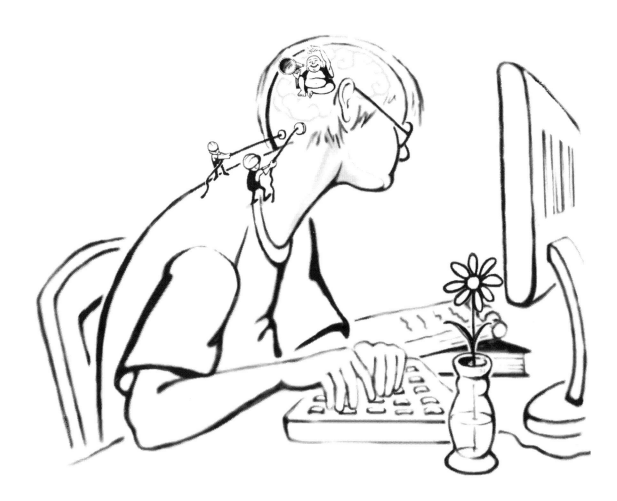

**FIGURE 2.5 NATURAL MUSCULAR COMPENSATION FOR
IMBALANCE:** During prolonged, one-sided tasks our brain is
constantly and silently monitoring where all of our parts are in
space so that we don't have to think about them. In the early
stage of compensation for mechanical imbalance, the brain
makes sure the right muscles work a little harder to keep us
from falling over.

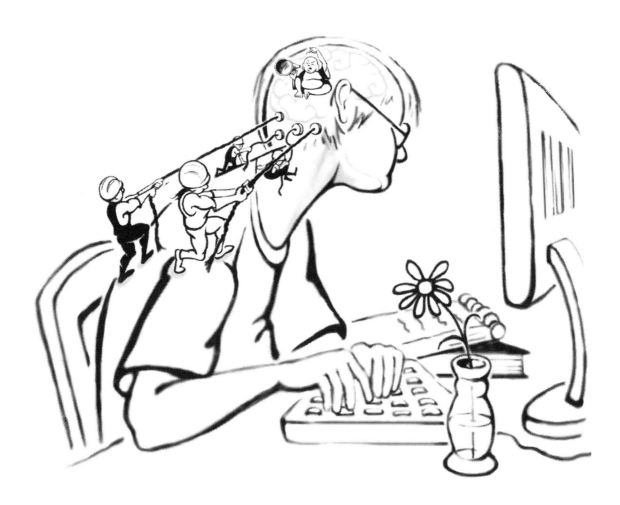

FIGURE 2.6 ELABORATE TISSUE COMPENSATION FROM PROLONGED ONE-SIDED TASKING: During later stages of compensation for one-sided tasking, it becomes time to recruit stronger neighboring muscles that normally are only designed for short, powerful bursts of activity.

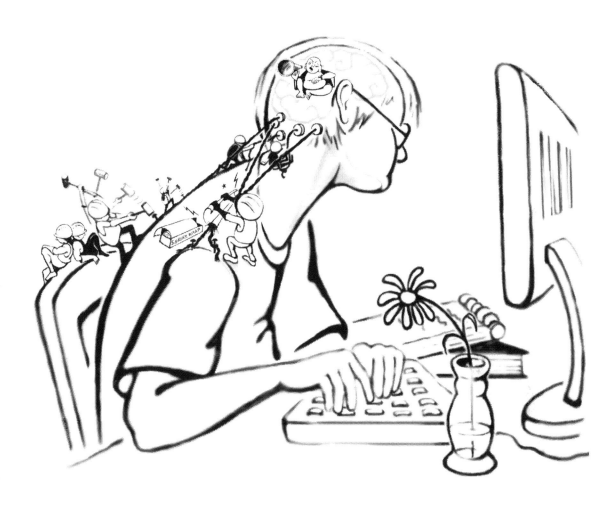

FIGURE 2.7 EXTREME MEASURES TO COPE WITH EXCESSIVE ONE-SIDED TASKING: Late-stage, one-sided tasking will lead to the formation of adhesions once other compensatory efforts are exhausted. Say goodbye to elasticity and hello to decreased flexibility and range of motion.

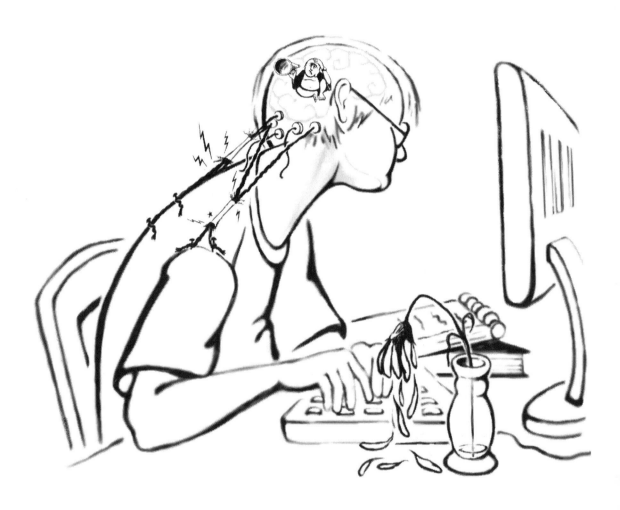

FIGURE 2.8 ADHESIONS—THE BEGINNING OF KNOTS: This is when sticky adhesions start to cause pain when we are doing the things we've done many times before.

Suffocated tissues aside, this tendency to adapt is at the heart of why we can go on for decades doing stressful things with our body outside of our individual, ideally safe neutral zone. We have no idea these things are actually biomechanically unsound because they don't hurt right away. We've adapted for quite some time by using our backup muscles. One of the most frequent comments I hear from patients is: "…but it never *used* to hurt to do _____ before!" Let's see how these ideas apply in the case of one of the patients I mentioned earlier.

What else was filling Ed's inflammation "bucket" to the brim?

As alarmed as Ed was by the pain from his reaching-for-the-toothbrush injury, by that point in the day he was exhausted and just decided to go lie down, hoping he'd wake up and it would all make sense again. He ended up going to sleep but was rudely reminded in the middle of the night while trying to turn over in bed that the pain was still with him. Getting up out of bed in the morning took even more negotiation and premeditation. He loosened up a bit in the shower and then more as he moved around the house. Since then, however, he feels like he is "hobbling" around, unable to straighten easily, especially after sitting. Sitting in the car on the way to work feels uncomfortable and hurts when he goes over rough pavement. Standing for long periods of time, like he has to do at work, makes him notice that his pain is more left sided and goes into the buttock and thigh on that side.

Ed is very frustrated by the intensity of this pain and how much it's affecting his ability to just go through his day. He also doesn't have patience for all the modifications his pain is forcing him to make. It's slowing down his work and making him cranky. He is worried that something is seriously wrong with him—after all, he's thinking there must be something really defective about his back for this sort of pain to come from simply standing and reaching for a tube of toothpaste! He recalls decades of hard labor associated with his carpentry that didn't cause any problems, and he feels he is a generally fit individual who is well within a healthy body mass index and reasonably active. He is an avid bicyclist and has done yoga and will still do some at home on his own when he has time—although, admittedly, since the birth of his second child, he has had very little time.

During Ed's treatment with me in the office, I was able to reintroduce some balance to the spine and pelvis and his body was very responsive. His tissues are healthy—he's right about the fact that he is generally a fit person, which is definitely working in his favor to get him back on track from this injury sooner rather than later. We talked a little more about how this isn't actually such an unreasonable reaction and that I often see these sorts of injuries that seem to come from minor movements around the house. Sitting on the couch for too long, sleeping in the wrong position for too long, washing dishes and loading the dishwasher—all of these things can trigger serious pain if the body has been working hard and is being pushed to the edge of its tolerance for any particular repetitive motion or activity.

At this point in our conversation, Ed remembers that earlier that day there was something a little out of the ordinary at work that he didn't think much of at the time, but now he realizes that this may have played a role in the downward spiral of that evening. He moves large pieces of carpentry all the time and is usually doing it with great planning and good form and with help from others, but this day there was something a buddy of his was trying to move and Ed decided to help. It turns out this was a deceptively heavy piece of carpentry as well as awkwardly shaped. At one point during the move, the piece slipped and would have fallen, had it not been for a quick maneuver on Ed's part. He now remembers that this was quite a bit more of a physical effort than he'd planned on or prepared for, and he may have sacrificed good-lifting technique for the sake of keeping the piece from falling. He didn't feel any sharp pain at the time and so didn't think much of it, but now he sees how that may have been a trigger and admits he did feel something in his back when it happened, but was able to just shrug it off.

It's not uncommon for me to learn during the course of treatment, and sometimes much later, about the real contributing stressors to a patient like Ed's pain. It often turns out that these may have been adding up for days, weeks or even years prior to the manifestation of that injury—suddenly bringing the bucket to the brim and setting it up to overflow at the slightest next move. These are important pieces of information, but once we understand that there is a reasonable cause for our pain, we are best served by focusing on how to control the smaller and less traumatic day-to-day triggers. Once we identify and eliminate the repetitive stressors of our routines at home or at work, the result can be transformative and, what was once thought to be pain we would just have to live with can be completely avoided going forward. Of course, these daily stressors can be steeped in habit and are not always so easily modified. When patients fall back into old habits is when they show up in my office in pain again.

The first time we experience failure of our structural back-up mechanisms, it can be very hard to accept that sometimes we simply have reached the limit of our adaptive capabilities and are left with no other option than to change the behavior that may have led us to that point in the first place—no matter how familiar that behavior may be. The performance and resilience of our backup mechanisms depend largely on overall body strength and elasticity, as well as general organ system effectiveness at clearing caustic byproducts *out* and allowing nutrients to flood *in*.

It follows, then, that people who keep up their overall body tone and fitness level are more likely to be able to get away with compromised structure and function than people who have less tone and thereby less muscular resilience. How is that, exactly? Muscle tissue provides elasticity. The more elastic something is, the more forgiving it is for deviations from neutral, and the more quickly it can "spring" back to neutral or its original shape—given the chance. Muscle activity (by repeated contract-relax motion) also provides mechanical pumping action to networks of vessels responsible for transport of nutrients and waste products, thereby helping the process. Remember, the less that waste is allowed to accumulate, the less chance we have of feeling the pain of inflammation.

The body's pre-programmed position of greatest ease has a lot to do with the original structural design of the spine. The spine is very specifically engineered to best support us in this shape (Figure 2.9).

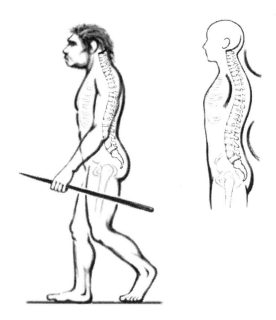

FIGURE 2.9 ORIGINAL SPINAL DESIGN: There is an optimal shape for the human spine that is designed to provide the best shock absorption possible and the least muscular strain in our upright movement against gravity. This optimal shape depends very much on the three main curves that you see in this image. When we lose these curves because of misinformation and bad habits, we become more vulnerable to mechanical stress and pain.

These curves, in combination with the shape of the bones, develop and stack the way they do for optimal body stability and shock absorption in the upright position. Any position or prolonged activity that forces even the slightest change in the shape of these curves will eventually result in compromise to the stability of the spine.

In turn, no matter how slight, this deviation from what our brain is programmed to consider neutral will trigger protective and corrective compensatory muscular reactions (Figure 2.10A-D).

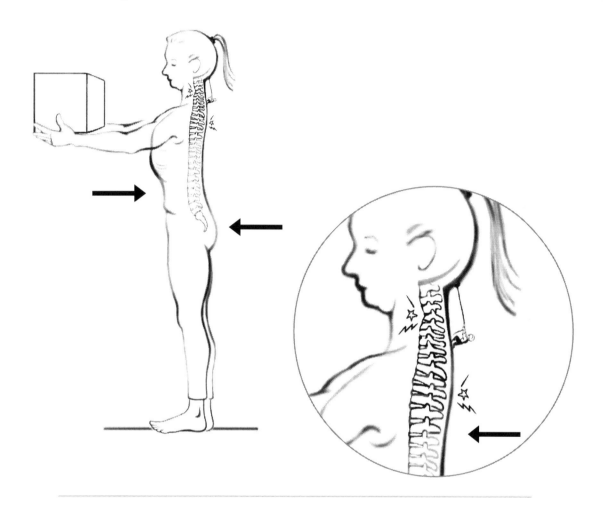

FIGURE 2.10A BACK BRACING GONE AWRY: Very commonly we brace the back by tucking the butt and sucking in the gut, thinking this is the right thing to do, but look what happens at the upper back and neck as a result. The loss of the naturally protective lower back curve/sway causes a stressful equal and opposite reaction in the spine.

CLOSE-UP: When we lose the appropriate curve in the mid back, we force the neck into an unnatural position and this triggers a stress response from the muscles of the neck as they try to correct and protect.

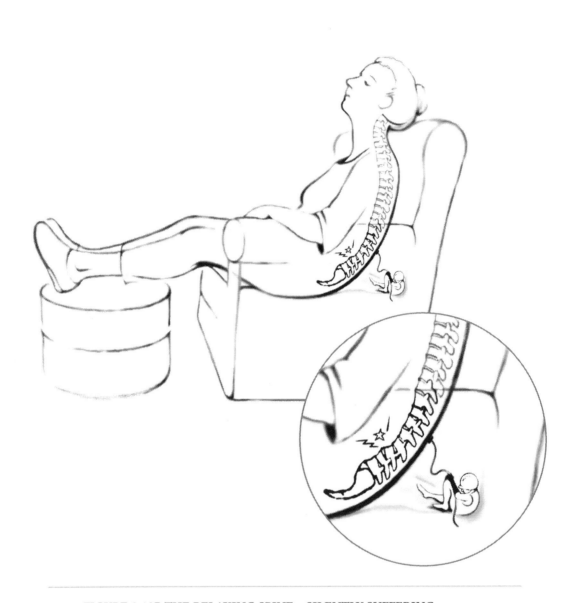

FIGURE 2.10B THE RELAXING SPINE—SILENTLY SUFFERING COMPRESSION AND BREEDING "LAZY" MUSCLES: When you think you're relaxing, you might be doing damage and causing compression. Compression while resting like this triggers the protective deactivation of spinal stabilizers, which teaches the back muscles to be lazy.

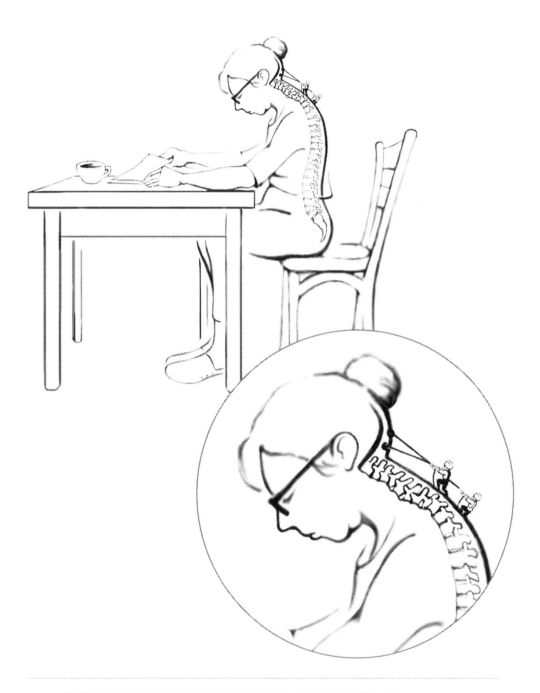

FIGURE 2.10C SEATED READING HEAD POSITIONING: Nice lower back curve, but look at how off-center (forward-leaning) the head is. No problem for short periods of time, but the upper back muscles are forced to work hard as they struggle to keep balance in an unbalanced situation.

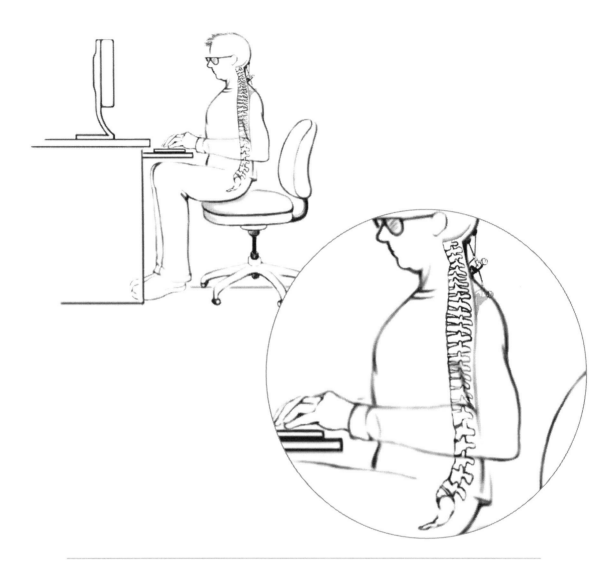

FIGURE 2.10D SEATED POSTURE THAT "LOOKS" GOOD ISN'T NECESSARILY GOOD FOR YOU: Looks like good posture, but see how the spine actually suffers to create this appearance: (1) Sucking the belly in forces the low back to curve the wrong way; (2) Squeezing shoulder blades together forces the mid back spine to flatten; and (3) Tucking the chin forces the neck to tip dangerously forward. This is the perfect recipe for stressing all the muscles of the spine in a way that can sneak up on us after years of doing so without pain. Good posture allows muscles to relax—bones are stacked optimally according to design as in Figure 2.9.

Notice how our body's deviations from neutral are handled by our brain like a mathematical equation. For as many pounds of pressure we shift forward, our spine shifts the exact same amount backward. For as many pounds of pressure we shift to one side, the spine shifts the same amount to the other side. Any time you see someone of advanced age stooped and bent in unexpected directions, what you are seeing is the result from years of playing this balancing game.

Again, our system can adapt for years before we realize we've been operating under suboptimal conditions. One thing important to note here is that asymmetry does not necessarily equal pain. It's the degree of *effort* or work spent trying to bring the body back to neutral once we stray from center that really matters. If that effort exceeds our capacity, then we have a recipe for pain, but not until that point. For some bodies, when they deviate from center, it looks noticeably crooked and for others it does not.[3] So it follows that pain is *not* necessarily the result of asymmetry. It *is*, however, most certainly the result of an uneven distribution of *work* being performed by the tissues of the body in an attempt to maintain balance. This means that spending energy trying to appear less crooked in an effort to alleviate pain can be a completely misguided waste of effort without first giving thought to our individual neutral zone. Becoming free of everyday pain must begin with finding a way to return to our unique neutral zone and understanding how to avoid deviating from it in the future. This is what you'll find more specific help with in *Volume Two: Fix the Fire Damage* and *Volume Three: Plan For Fire Prevention.*

Deviation from neutral positioning results in *muscular tightening*, which can be the *cause* or it can be the *result* of an inflammatory reaction. So, you'll never find one without the other. If you've ever received a massage when you're feeling well, you know that muscular tightness can exist without pain—that is, at least until someone therapeutically touches those muscles and then we realize we've been walking around all wound up but without necessarily feeling anything uncomfortable. Only when this tightness is accompanied by the irritation of inflammation do we begin to notice the existing muscle tightness without any outside prompting.

Often, the pain of inflammation is accompanied by a muscular reaction referred

---

3. There are individual congenital variances to bone symmetry that can make one person's neutral zone appear visually more crooked than another's who may not have such anatomical bony asymmetry.

to as "splinting." Splinting is when muscles tighten in an effort to protect by preventing movement—just like the splint you would wear if you sprained a finger. The irony is that splinting, over time, can also initiate or lead to more inflammation because it is only partially successful at limiting motion. This means the remaining range of motion is now happening in the presence of resistance as the splinting hugs all the nearby structures closer to each other. This resistance causes friction and this increased friction is what can cause tissue irritation to the point of painful inflammation. So here we have what can be a vicious cycle of pain that many of us have trouble finding our way out of or making any sense of (Diagram 2.1).

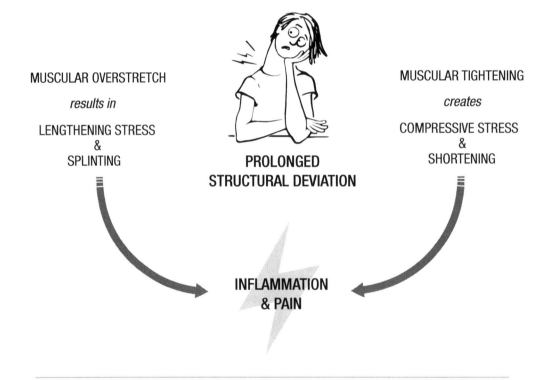

DIAGRAM 2.1 PROLONGED STRUCTURAL DEVIATION: Some of the seemingly benign positions we find ourselves in during the course of a regular day can be causing and reinforcing our pain and inflammation.

The other and much under-recognized mechanical cause of inflammation-related pain is *excessive movement*. Excessive movement, or joint hyper-mobility, is something that can exist body-wide or in just a few areas. It can be the result of injury or it can be a genetic predisposition and a function of our biochemical make-up. Available movement at any given joint is largely a function of friction or space between bones, ligament tone and muscular flexibility. Hyper-mobility is usually due to loss of tone or tension at the ligaments, which are like guide wires that hold our bones together. We don't always know that we have

> "Pain is *not* necessarily the result of asymmetry."

this condition, and those who do are often surprised to learn of it, especially because it is typically accompanied by the overwhelming sensation of tight muscles. The overwhelming muscle tightness in this case is a smart protective adaptation. It is that protective splinting reaction referred to in Diagram 2.1, but on a larger scale. When this kind of protective muscle tension is alleviated by massage or stretching, the underlying problem is uncovered and pain can actually increase.

The idea of "excessive" motion most likely provokes images of circus performers, and, yes, these people are prime candidates for this problem; but, because they are usually so strong and well conditioned, they will not fully suffer from the effects of it until they transition to a more sedentary lifestyle. Hyper-mobility can take us outside of our pre-programmed acceptable neutral zone repeatedly and precariously (according to the brain's pre-programmed set points) with our everyday movements. We can only expect that for safety's sake the nervous system, relying on its blueprint for survival, will find a way to compensate for that by initiating protective mechanisms. In the spirit of protection, repetitive excessive motion can cause adjacent ("neighboring") areas—joints and muscles—to lock up in an attempt to stabilize. But the opposite can happen as well. When we go for years with compromised areas of the spine that have protectively locked up for other reasons, the adjacent areas (sometimes spinal joints and sometimes joints and muscles farther from the spine) in *that* case have to pick up slack and become excessively mobile to compensate for the areas that have stopped functioning at full range (Figure 2.11).

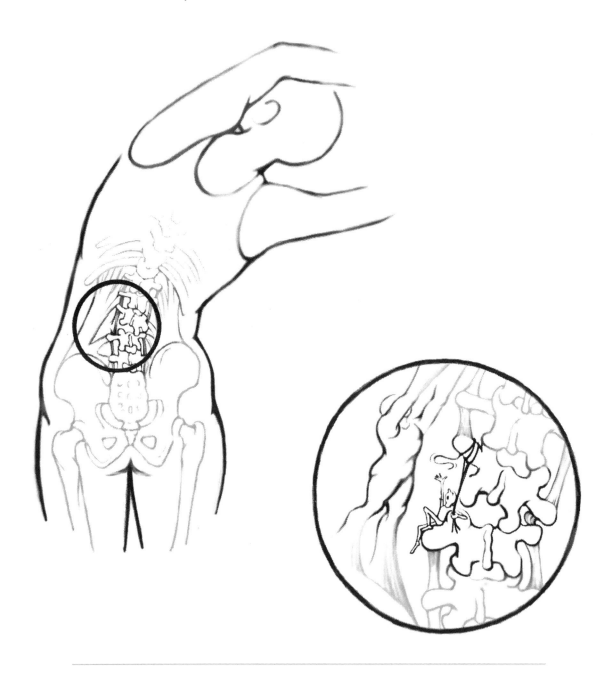

FIGURE 2.11 THE RESULT OF LIGAMENT LAXITY: When the ligaments are too loose to do the job of stabilizing, the larger muscle groups are left with the work of over-engaging in order to do the stabilizing work needed. This is why so often people who have hyper-mobile joints struggle with the deceiving sensation of tightness and the craving for stretch.

No matter what the cause (genetic or regional), cases of hyper-mobility are likely to result in signs of inflammation because of movement that repeatedly exceeds the normal range that the joint structure and neighboring tissues were designed to sustain.[i] Again we have inflammation—this time from too much movement (rather than prolonged, one-sided leaning postures)—and muscle splinting now is the *result* instead of the cause or trigger for all of it. The more the muscles splint, guard and tighten, the more irritation there is to the body as it goes about daily activity, and sooner or later we will be notified of this compensatory imbalance by the appearance of pain. Pain means we have reached the end of our compensatory capabilities.

> "Moving two attached objects away from each other will always stress the connection between them."

Many people who enjoy easy flexibility for most of their lives are the ones who suffer from the most confusing kinds of pain syndromes. Flexibility is widely associated with good function and health, but, when there is a lifetime of this sort of excessive movement, the absence of stability is often overlooked until injury ensues. The challenge of stabilizing a body like this is great and the inflammatory response can be very difficult to control once begun. Let's look at how this happened in one of those cases mentioned earlier.

When being limber becomes too much of a good thing

CHARLENE, that 32-year-old modern dancer and yoga instructor who came to see me for help with the stabbing mid-back pain, is also a new mom. While she was pregnant, she saw me for low back and mid-back pain that seemed to develop as her body changed with the pregnancy, which is very common. She responded very well, and, like most pregnant patients, it didn't take much to relieve her joint restrictions. Because of the loosening effect of pregnancy hormones on the ligaments and other soft tissues of the body, I don't need to use a whole lot of force to encourage things to move the right way again. It's something I see a lot, and so didn't think anything of it with Charlene when I was treating her during this time.

Fast forward to 18 months later, Charlene is complaining of this sudden, stabbing mid-back and chest pain that took her breath away—all while simply walking from her car to the store with nothing more than her purse, sensibly slung diagonally over her shoulders and pushing the stroller. It turns out to be a sprain at one of the joints between the rib and the spine where the rib meets with the mid-back, and it's causing her torso to freeze up with painful muscle spasms. She returned to teaching yoga 5 weeks after her son was born, and now she is back to rehearsing for a dance performance that will be happening in a few months. She is still breast feeding and, since this mid-back pain started, breast feeding positions are extremely uncomfortable. She has to remain rigid in order to avoid the shooting pain, and now her muscles are so tight they are causing quite a persistent ache even if she does remain rigid. The only relief she gets is by lying down.

After some time on the treatment table, Charlene adds that she has been noticing extraordinary leg tightness down the back of both legs. It seems to her there is no amount of hamstring stretching she can do to alleviate this tightness. She seems able to dance without that sensation, but when she is warming up beforehand it's very apparent to her how tight the backs of her legs are. And because this is so different for her from before the arrival of her son, she has just come to accept that the tightness is from her de-conditioning during pregnancy. When I tested her hamstrings with the straight leg raise leg lift while she was lying on her back, I easily reached a 90-degree range of motion and then some—easy flexibility true to a dancer's body. Charlene reported no pain or tightness with my stretch of her hamstrings, until I took her leg even higher, bringing her knee almost to her face. Her body complied, but in order to accomplish this the lower back has to start rounding, and that is when she did feel a touch of the hamstring tightness. She explains the tightness is something she notices when she is warming up for dance or just going about taking care of her daily activities.

Upon further observation it becomes apparent to me that this patient has lost structural stability in her lower back—especially when she is sitting; the lower back collapses into a rounded position—despite perfectly good hamstring flexibility by most people's standards. Every movement she makes to care for her son involves reaching and bending forward, all of which occurs with her lower back (probably inadvertently) rounding forward. This rounding was not apparent during her pregnancy because of how the weight of her belly pulled her lower back into an appropriate arch or "sway." She is not having lower back pain these days, but the spine is not designed to be rounded in this area and, in order to cope, the areas above and below end up grabbing on in an effort to stabilize the big picture and attempt to relieve the lower back of an unnatural stress. Rounding in an area where it's not supposed to happen causes irritation due to friction near the openings in the spine between vertebrae through which nerves thread themselves in order to feed into the leg muscles—in this case, the hamstrings. This is what is giving her the sensation of tightness without actual tightness by structural standards. It's the excessive motion in her spine that is making her feel tight legs—a classic presentation for the dancer's body.

Additionally, this repeated excessive rounding in the lower back is not within the safe neutral zone of movement, and so her brain has assigned extra work to the muscles of her mid-back, which have been doing their best to compensate for the excess movement by splinting (refer to Diagram 2.1). It turns out that just before her mid-back spasm occurred she was reaching (as she's done countless times by now) into the back seat of the car to get her son out of his car seat, lifting him out and into the stroller. Undoubtedly, the lower back rounded forward as it usually does, but today was just one too many times, which caused the mid-back to react protectively. This all makes good sense to me but can feel confusing for the body it's happening to because of the widespread misconception that flexibility is always good—combined with the memory of doing this same thing many times without injury. We have to be careful how we measure and judge flexibility. Too much of any good thing can definitely be trouble, and flexibility into the wrong directions is quite a bit of trouble.

CHAPTER 3

Chemical Triggers of Everyday Pain

INJURY OR STRESS OF A CHEMICAL nature occurs when an area is overwhelmed with cellular waste or byproducts. There is a normal constant flow of cellular waste as the result of our daily metabolic activity. Just as we eat, drink and go to the bathroom on a daily basis, our cells are doing the same thing on a microscopic level. A backup of these waste byproducts can happen during inflammation because of a mechanical tissue injury as previously mentioned, but waste products can also accumulate without any physical injury, at all. This build-up can happen if there is either: (1) Too much cellular waste being produced too quickly;[4] or (2) Elimination of cellular waste is somehow compromised or too slow. Both of these things can happen when the body's critical biochemical and metabolic processes are being stressed (causing more waste or garbage to result and accumulate) and/or if the

---

4. Occasionally the body has more "trash" to break down and get rid of. Allergens, viruses, and toxins in the environment can add to the "trash" load in our system.

body's elimination organs and systems are bogged down and sluggish (slowing down the movement of garbage *out* of the body).

Examples of what can add to the production of cellular waste are allergens, toxins and other environmental or dietary stressors. How much of a burden the body considers these to be varies from person to person, but we're all handling some degree of biochemical stress as a natural result of living. While it's a given that we're all dealing with some amount of metabolic burden, if it becomes a noticeable problem (by the expression of pain or inflammation), more often than not there is likely a deficit on the clean-up side of the equation. Clean-up capacity (our ability to rid our body of chemical stressors or irritants) is controlled in part by *physical activity*, which creates a pumping motion (or exerts an external massaging action) that pushes things along. Control of clean-up is also assisted by *hydration*—drinking water exerts internal hydraulic pressure on the vessels to help them flush the trash out. Still another part of clean-up is made possible by *enzymes* that the body makes and that we also can take in through our diet. Enzymes are the body's molecular construction workers. There are demolition-crew enzymes to take big molecules apart and there are building-contractor enzymes to assemble molecules and make all sorts of chemical processes run smoothly. Preparing waste for elimination requires the demolition enzymes to break it down into manageable and more benign bits. Elimination organs and systems of the body include everything from the colon, kidneys, the lymphatic system[5] and the skin (Figure 3.1).

Knowing that these three factors (movement, hydration and enzyme action) are primarily responsible for driving clean-up of molecular waste, and that build-up of molecular waste is one thing that can cause inflammation and pain, then we can say that two ways to intentionally influence or expedite this clean-up to ease the chemical burden on the tissues is through diet (hydration and intake of enzymes) and exercise (movement). Now, isn't that a tired old idea, diet and exercise?! Yes, but one to take to heart, and as you read on about chemical triggers maybe you'll gain a better appreciation of how powerful these two timeless tools are.

---

5. Lymph is the colorless fluid of the lymphatic system, which consists of a network of vessels containing white blood cells designed to drain the body tissues of waste and foreign invaders like allergens, viruses and bacteria, among others. Lymph flows from the tissue spaces to the bloodstream as it cleans things up. Lymph nodes are the little stations along that network that act as microscopic sewage treatment plants.

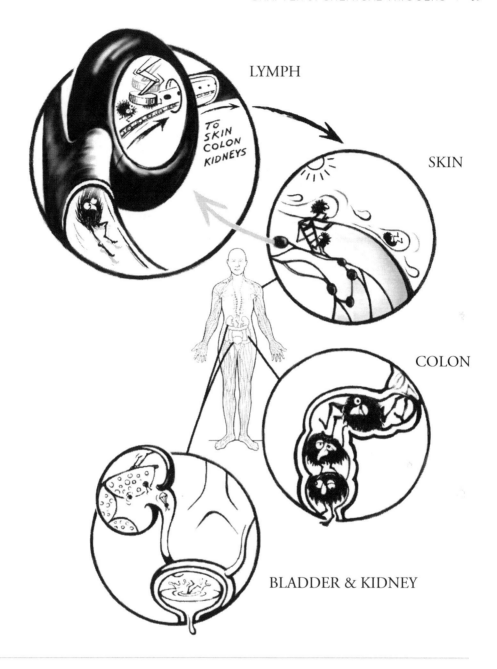

FIGURE 3.1 ORGANS AND SYSTEMS OF ELIMINATION: These are the organs and systems busy escorting waste byproducts out of the body every minute of every day, making sure garbage gets out. The lymphatic network of nodes, vessels and fluid wash tissue clean and launch immune responses to neutralize the trash. Skin allows the escape of molecules via sweat. The colon escorts less useful, solid waste out. Kidneys and bladder are carefully allowing passage of filtered liquids.

> "Just like the blueprint that outlines our body's ideal *mechanical* position, there is also a *chemical* 'ideal.'"

When dealing with pain anywhere in the body, we should keep in mind how much of an impact we can have on our recovery by paying attention to some of the main things we can control, which are nutrients, hydration and movement. Even if the pain you're having is in your little toe, your body chemistry impacts all of it. The next two volumes in this series (*Volume Two: Fix the Fire Damage*, and *Volume Three: Plan For Fire Prevention*) will both tackle specific components of how we can use nutrients and movement techniques to strike a better chemical balance along with physical balance while remembering that the management of the chemical balance plays just as much (if not more) of a role in bolstering against re-injury as does physical strengthening.

pH—Our Acid/Base Balance

Just like the blueprint that outlines our body's ideal *mechanical* position (for providing the least amount of muscular effort while maintaining optimal organ housing), there is also a *chemical* "ideal" set-point at which there is greatest biological efficiency or potential and least likelihood of inflammation and disease. pH levels, or the balance between acid and base in the body, is the measure by which this chemical set point is evaluated. The ideal pH range for lymph (clean-up crew) and body tissues (*extra*-cellular[6] space, where all the clean-up happens) is 7.8 to 8.0, which is on the alkaline side of things (opposite from acidic). If all systems are operating optimally, then this alkaline tissue pH value makes us naturally resistant to the many microbes that

---

6. "Extra"cellular means outside of the cells but still in the tissue space, thus in contrast with "intra"cellular, which means inside of the cells.

are happier in an acid environment, like some bacteria. For example, *Streptococcus* (responsible for things like strep throat, impetigo, scarlet fever) or *Staphylococcus aureus* (responsible for skin infections, and some food poisoning) thrives best at pH levels on the acidic side of the scale (6.7–7.5).[ii]

This is just one example of how important pH in different systems of the body can be. For optimal functioning of *all* systems, the pH of our tissues (*extra*cellular pH) generally needs to be on the alkaline side to allow proper cellular functioning. Think about how water boils best at a certain temperature (usually 100 degrees Celsius) at sea level atmospheric pressure. Well, similarly, the millions of chemical reactions that need to happen for the proper break-down of waste to occur, all operate best at this less acidic (more alkaline) pH range (*extra*cellular pH).

On the other hand, the ideal pH for blood (*intra*cellular pH) is naturally a bit more acidic than that of tissue but still technically on the alkaline side overall at 7.4 to 7.46. The pH of blood has *very* little room for error. In fact, the successful functioning of our heart depends on keeping within this extremely strict parameter. A blood pH outside of this tight range is actually life threatening.[iii] Because of this very specific requirement by the blood, acid–base balance of the body becomes an extremely important and delicate balancing act. Because *blood* (*intra*cellular) pH *must* be maintained within this narrow range at all costs and at all times, pH levels in other parts of the body (*extra*cellular) will be compromised in order to make that happen.

Parents of little children can relate to this dynamic: Imagine that a happy or sleeping baby represents the perfect blood pH level. Mom and Dad or other care-givers are pH levels elsewhere in the body. If that baby is crying, or unhappy in any way, these caregivers will do whatever it takes to make that baby happy again—even if it means sacrificing their own sleep or happiness—for the sake of the overall peace in the house. When that baby (blood) pH is unhappy, the optimal functioning of the household (body tissue and salivary pH) is thrown off. When Mom and Dad tend to that baby to restore the happy pH, functioning is restored but with some compromise to the caregiver pH (e.g., maybe stressed shoulders from holding and rocking the child to sleep or becoming sleep deprived themselves). But with happy baby pH balance, other essential daily tasks can resume.

Saliva is a component of a body system (digestion) that will show compromise to its own pH levels when overall balance is at risk. Salivary pH needs to be on the acidic side (6.4–6.8) in order to assist properly in the first stages of digestion and to act as the first line of defense against many viruses, should we happen to put something in our mouth that a virus latched on to (which, unlike bacteria, generally doesn't survive well in acidic environments). But, if push comes to shove, the pH of saliva will yield to the pressure and take the hit by becoming less acidic just to keep the blood pH level where it needs to be within its very rigid parameters.

Stress causes a real chemical reaction that floods the body tissues with substances known to be acidifying. Many aspects of the modern diet—heavy in starches and meats and refined sugars—also have an acidifying effect on the body. In order to keep these acidifying factors from affecting our delicate blood pH (happy baby), the body goes into regulating mode and the compromising "caregiver" systems take a hit. Parts that can afford to (extracellular pH = most body tissues except blood) will take on the acid onslaught rather than let the blood feel any of the acidifying effect. In response to this, other areas like saliva, which are *supposed* to be more acidic, have to become alkaline to keep the overall balance—and so we lose some of our digestive ability and defenses against invaders.

When our internal lymph fluids and tissue or "extracellular" pH levels are pushed into a less ideal acidic state, it forces the normally protective acidic salivary pH to shift the other way and it becomes more alkaline and less protective against those upper respiratory viruses. To avoid this shift toward more alkaline and therefore less protective saliva (in conjunction with more acidic body tissues), it takes a conscious effort on our part at these three things:

1. Clean diet
2. Moderate exercise
3. Stress management

All three of these factors when neglected or unregulated tend to have acidifying effects on the internal tissues of the body. These are all the hazards of modern life (poor food choices, stress and lack of physical activity). Unfortunately, it's these daily common hazards that can easily lead to a shift in our acid–base balance for the worse: more acidic tissues lead to more alkaline saliva (Diagram 3.1A and Diagram 3.1B).[7]

Why on earth are we talking so much about pH? Here's the clincher: research shows that acid pH in the body tissues is a key aspect associated with pain and inflammation.[iv] Where there is acidity, there is potential for pain!

All of the substances released by and around injured tissue to help with repair are actually acidifying molecules! This is one of the main reasons there is pain when parts of our body are stressed and injured. Of course when we break a bone there is pain because a structure, rich with sensitive nerve endings has been mechanically disrupted or traumatized, but the pain that can continue long after the trauma has been dealt with is because of the biochemistry playing out behind the scenes.

Here are the facts you need to know:

1. Cellular waste of healthy tissues is naturally acidic
2. Injured tissues break down into acidic molecules
3. The repair response itself releases acidic molecules

So, if acidity in the tissues is associated with pain, then this explains why pain can be the result when any one of these three things is going on. Based on the three aforementioned facts, we can safely say that tissue acidity levels are on the rise whenever there is stress or injury, as the result of a repair effort in progress, or when healthy tissues are simply living and breathing, so to speak, because the result of routine tissue metabolism is the production of an acidic cellular waste. This is why so often it doesn't make any obvious sense to us why we have pain. It's all happening behind the scenes as part of a chemical balancing act we can't see until it falls suddenly out of balance. Recall that inflammation (at the heart of all pain) is the result of a traffic-jam–style build-up of a combination of normal waste products and repair molecules (Figure 3.2B).

---

7. There are complexities to the physiologic pH levels that this book will not be able to do justice to, but further reading is encouraged. Refer to the index for more information.

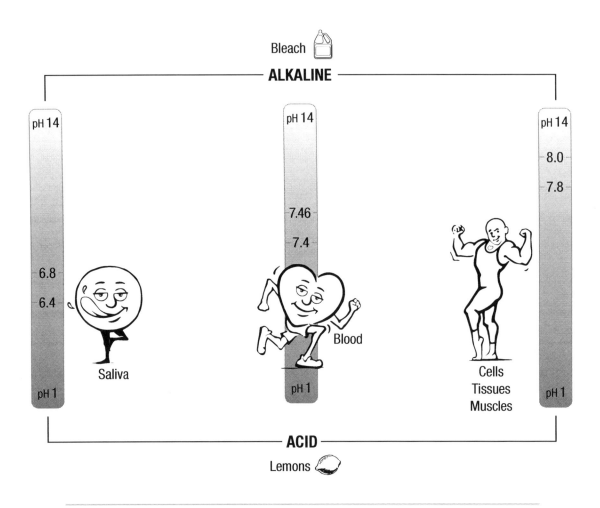

DIAGRAM 3.1A IDEAL ACID–ALKALINE RELATIONSHIP BETWEEN SALIVA, BLOOD AND BODY TISSUES: Each one's success depends on the other two.

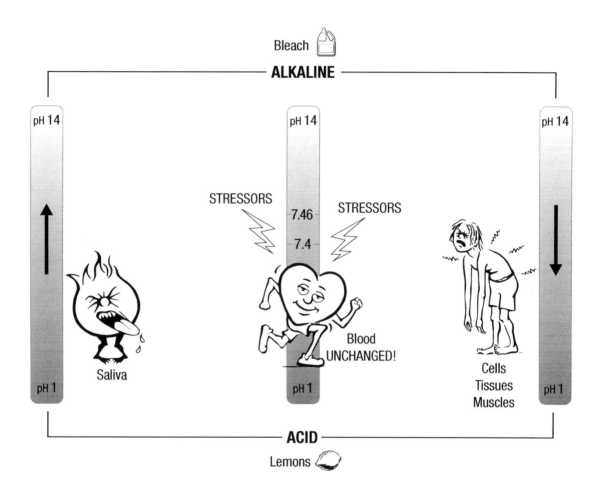

DIAGRAM 3.1B ACID–ALKALINE LEVELS OUT OF BALANCE:
Stressors that cause this imbalance come from tissue injury,
intake of suboptimal food, air and water as well as emotional
strain. All of these things are acidifying. Maintaining slightly
alkaline pH of blood is paramount. Saliva and tissue pH will
become compromised in order to compensate for imbalance.
Saliva becomes more alkaline and tissues become more acidic.

Now, if a person's system is generally more acidic to start with, maybe as a result of lifestyle (stress and diet), genetics or disease, then just imagine how much *more* of an impact it can have when he or she experiences any kind of additional tissue stressors. There is simply not much room left for error, just like in my patient Ed's case.

"Ouch, my pH!"

Our pal **ED** keeps feeling more and more confident about his lower back as time goes by and he continues to pay attention to his everyday habits—trying to avoid stressing his spine as much as is realistically possible for him— and now I've been able to move on to assigning him daily strengthening exercises specific to his issue. Interestingly, during his most recent visit, he recalls during our conversation that around the same time as his lower back gave out he was at his highest daily coffee intake and in fact was struggling with stomach pain a few days before his back gave way. He had good intentions of decreasing the coffee, but until his back injury happened, he wasn't able to commit to it. The back pain motivated him to do more good things for himself and try to minimize pain everywhere, so he has cut back since then but is flirting with a second cup in the afternoon again more recently.

What catches my attention about this information regarding the coffee-related stomach pain is the fact that coffee is indisputably a pH game changer. It's extremely acidifying and therefore can be a significant contributing inflammatory trigger for some people. Many of us are able to manage a cup here and there without flying into a crisis and it certainly can have benefits, which, for some people, might outweigh the drawbacks. But when the body is stressed already, like Ed's was, the increasingly massive amounts of coffee were probably part of what pushed him to the edge and made it so easy for his body to react to what, for him, would normally have been a tiny mechanical trigger. The stomach pain is a sign that there was already an inflammatory situation in that area of his body and it was only a matter of time before the neighboring structures became stressed by that (Figure 8.1).

After hearing this I urged Ed to keep the coffee intake as low as possible, and, because I know Ed also enjoys a microbrew at the end of the day, I explained that those two things together will set him up for another inflammatory event if he is not careful. I shared with him some ideas for offsetting the inflammatory effects of the coffee and beer by considering adding a daily anti-inflammatory herbal supplement like turmeric with enzymes to help his system deal with the inflammation load in the body and the whole pH balancing act.

Now, another aspect of this stomach pain caused by coffee is the fact that, if there was active pain around the upper abdomen for a few weeks, then there was very possibly some protective structural collapsing happening in this area. Can you picture what your posture might look like if you had a belly ache? Well, the instinct to curl into a ball in reaction to belly pain causes a tightening in the front of the body even if we don't give in to it. This simple tightening can start to throw off the front-to-back balancing act, and our back muscles start having a lot of extra work to do in order to counter-balance that forward pull created by the protective reflexes.

Mediators of Inflammation

The substances that show up in response to tissue stress signals are referred to as "mediators of inflammation" because they are there to facilitate ("mediate") the inflammation

> "Stress causes a real chemical reaction that floods the body tissues with substances known to be acidifying."

management response. Inflammatory mediators are essentially the "clean-up crew" in and around the area of stress (the treadmill in Figures 3.2A and 3.2B). As we saw in Chapter 1, one of the ways this clean-up crew manages inflammation is by creating vasodilation, which is the opening up of access pathways that lead to the area under stress (the hallway to and from the treadmill room). These mediators include a wide variety of molecular compounds (prostaglandins, substance P, cytokines, serotonin and leukotrienes are just a few). Some are produced by the liver. Others are released by the surrounding tissue via a complex cellular communication network initiated at the first sign of stress or injury. All of these substances are known to cause pain sensitivity due to their ability to lower pH—creating a more acid environment in the area of stress (remember that acidity in the body is a recipe for pain!). Unfortunately, inflammatory mediators on their own have been found to cause even *more* pain in an already acidic environment.[v] This seems a little like adding fuel to the fire, doesn't it? It also serves as another explanation of why keeping our body more alkaline and less acidic can help fight pain.

Think back to our original example: after a run on the treadmill (the *mechanical* trigger), we may still experience sore muscles and/or general fatigue a day or more later. This is due to the lingering *chemical* triggers of pain—which we sometimes perceive in the form of "stiffness" as well as soreness. (Take a look at Figure 3.2A and notice the lingering clean-up crew even after the treadmill stress stops.)

An important fact emerges: chemical irritation by any acidifying molecules can also exist, all on its own—without any mechanical stress trigger at all. This can happen if the processes responsible for keeping normal everyday traffic moving in and around any one area become compromised in any way and a back-up were to result (take a look now at Figure 3.2B and notice the traffic jam in the absence of any treadmill stress).

Some of the well-meaning inflammatory mediator substances themselves (like prostaglandins, substance P and cytokines), while assisting with clean-up, are actually known to increase our sensitivity to pain! The sooner we can flush them away, the better. No disrespect to them and their ominous task of controlling inflammation, but they quickly outstay their welcome!

There is one mediator in particular (substance P) that, while pitching in during clean-up, will cause the release of the *dreaded* cyclo-oxygenase-2 (COX-2) enzymes. You might recognize the name "COX-2" from the widely marketed anti-inflammatory medications known for being "COX-2 *inhibitors.*" This is because COX-2 enzymes are not very welcome guests. They, in turn, cause the release of *more* gangs of pain-causing compounds (prostaglandins), which directly cause pain all on their own, and yet both are natural results of inflammation—an otherwise helpful process for cleaning up after injury.[8,vi] It should be pointed out that the introduction of COX-2 into the picture only occurs when inflammation has become a chronic situation. Whenever reasonably possible, it is key to find out what your pain triggers are and to avoid them as soon as possible in order to skip waking up these pain-causing COX-2 enzymes.[9]

An interesting example of the interplay between body chemistry and pain is a woman's body postpartum. There are a lot of chemical changes throughout pregnancy, and some of those changes linger for quite some time after delivery and throughout the breastfeeding year(s). There's very good reason for all of those changes and ligamentous laxity—a loosening of all the connective tissues of the body—is one of those useful changes. It's an essential feature to help facilitate the mechanics of childbirth, and, depending on each woman's individual chemical constitution and genetic make-up, this can sometimes linger long after the child is born.

---

8. COX-2 plays a helpful anti-inflammatory role in later stages of inflammation and it's possible that taking COX-2 inhibitors (e.g., celecoxib) will prolong inflammation, not cure it.

9. There are systemic conditions that can become chronic without much warning and then avoiding triggers will only lessen the pain, not completely eliminate it, which, in some cases, is the best we can hope for.

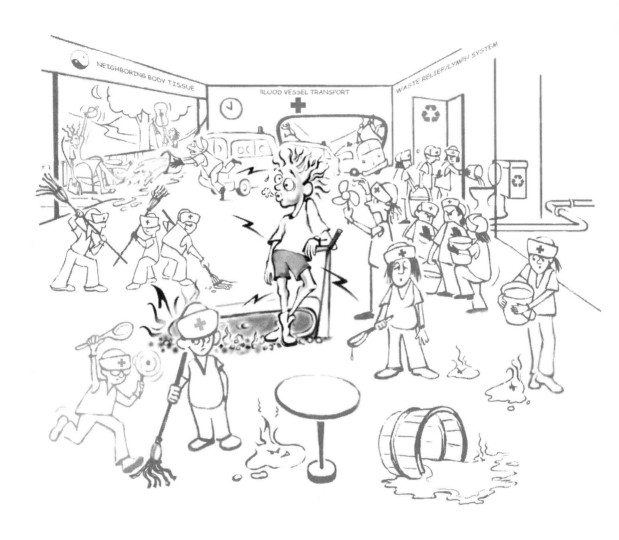

FIGURE 3.2A WHEN THE MECHANICAL STRESS STOPS: Even after the mechanical stress ceases, the chemical irritants (clean-up molecules and cellular waste products) can accumulate and linger long afterward. Inflammatory mediators ("helper molecules") can cause pain.

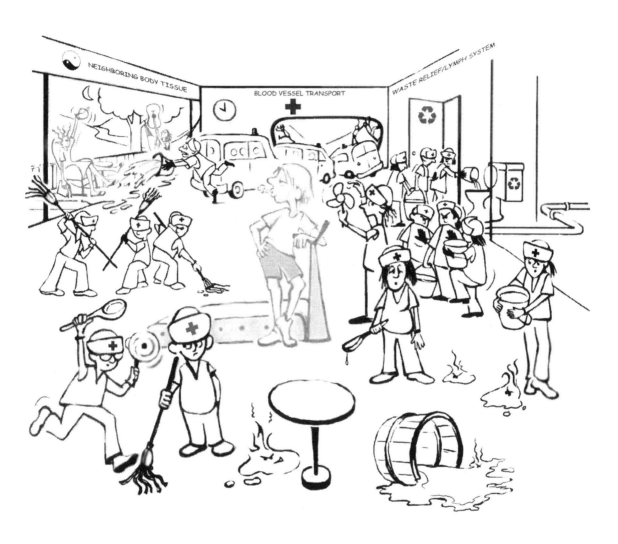

FIGURE 3.2B BUILD-UP OF EVEN THE HELPFUL INFLAMMATORY MEDIATORS CAN CAUSE PAIN: Long after mechanical stress or strain has ceased, we see chemical mediators of inflammation (clean-up crew) and natural cellular waste products are now building up and becoming crowded and cranky, as the demand for help increases. The ongoing production of cellular waste, in combination with a rising number of helper molecules on the scene, is now creating added tissue stress all of its own.

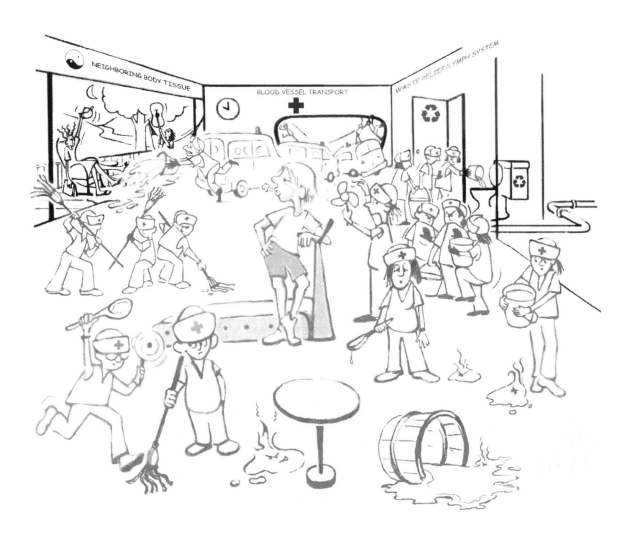

FIGURE 3.2C OVERCROWDING OF IRRITATING MOLECULES CAN CAUSE PAIN IN NEIGHBORING TISSUES: When the crowding of helper molecules and waste products is allowed to linger and grow, we have to start expecting that the neighboring tissues will begin suffering some of the spillover too! The neighboring body tissues, blood vessel transport and the waste relief/lymph system will all have an increased load to handle as balance is regained in the area while clean-up crew continues to clear out excess irritating molecules from the stressed or injured body part.

Charlene and her chemical recalibration after childbirth

Do you remember **CHARLENE'S** mid-back pain and spasm that came out of nowhere? It made a lot of sense to me when I saw how much her no-longer-pregnant lower back was rounding and collapsing forward compared to when she was pregnant (which is precisely what set her up for mid-back failure, as we saw). Even though this makes sense to me from a functional anatomy point of view, Charlene is left extremely frustrated that a simple and necessary movement like reaching into the car to get her son out of the car seat could have triggered this amount of alarming pain, and who can blame her? She's been putting her infant son in and taking him out of the car for three months now without a problem like this. I explained to her that, in addition to less-than-perfect biomechanics (rounding her lower back while reaching and bending into the car—not to mention her son's increasing weight), her body in particular is more vulnerable and therefore more unpredictably reactive. It's because of the excess mobility in her spine, firstly due to her life-long work with yoga and dance, but now especially that her body is post-pregnancy and still breastfeeding; her ligaments are even more lax than before she became pregnant.

At the end of this first visit to my office for her mid-back sprain, I learn that just last month Charlene started having her period again for the first time since giving birth and is possibly due to start her period again in the next week. This was yet another factor stacking against her during that instant when simply reaching into the back seat for her son resulted in unexpected sharp pain. It's been shown that, leading up to the period part of the menstrual cycle, necessary changes in hormones cause inflammation[vii] and ligament laxity. The ligaments are one of the main things holding our bones together and, when they get loose and wobbly because of an injury or chemical changes from pregnancy, the muscles are left in charge of holding things in the "right" place. Without the usual stability of the ligaments, the muscles often will overreact by grabbing on and clamping down—creating a sensation of tight and knotted muscles over time. Add inflammation to this mix and you have a bucket of pain brimming to the top and ready to overflow at the next slightest stress. So, even though Charlene is a limber, fit young woman with a high degree of tissue elasticity who would normally not have had to think twice about reaching into a car to get her son out of his car seat, on that particular day she had a number of chemical factors working against her in addition to some reasonable but repetitive mechanical stressors. Not only was this routine activity of putting her son in the stroller from the car seat, reaching its *mechanical* limit, but with the added *chemical* inflammation from her impending next menstrual period, plus the ligament laxity that commonly lingers in the body this soon after pregnancy (and for some women until they stop breastfeeding), poor Charlene had no chance against the ensuing mid-back and rib sprain that brought her into my office.

Stress Chemicals and Stress Addiction

"Addicted to stress?" You might be thinking: "…like a workaholic…?" Maybe a little bit, but stress addiction is not something you can easily see, and nobody will tell you that they *crave* more stress. No way. But some people will find themselves unable to shake stress no matter what they do. This is because it's so much deeper than a single simple behavior and it shouldn't be taken lightly. Your body actually has the capacity to become *chemically dependent* on the stress response in the same way that it can become dependent on any other substance or behavior—like food, alcohol or a gambling addiction, for example. We've come to accept that addictions are biologically based to a large degree and the perpetuating payoff is experienced physiologically—in the body—inside of our cells and brain. The same thing is true for stress addiction, but without the benefit of any consistent, identifiable external action or outward choice sending us into the reward phase. An alcoholic takes a drink. A food addict puts something into his or her mouth. A gambler places a bet. When we're addicted to *stress*, the body and brain are doing a neurochemical dance that is *invisible* to the naked eye, but the mechanism of addiction is exactly the same as it is with any other. Let's take a look.

> "Chemical irritation by any acidifying molecules can also exist, all on its own without any mechanical stress trigger."

By now you understand that our body's pH plays a very important role in everyday pain. Three main triggers that can cause a pH imbalance are food, activity levels and stress. Things that lead to a pH imbalance inside of our body tissues include the accumulation of everyday cellular waste as well as the mere presence of any molecules associated with the inflammation process (should there happen to be any), but the third trigger is *stress!* All of us have stress: the stress of work demands, moving to a new city, relationships ending, becoming a new parent or any number of such life changes. Well, guess what? All of these and many even lesser stressful life events also can make very real changes to your body chemistry and pH levels—chemical changes that can profoundly impact the degree of injury and recovery. They can lead you to be more susceptible to injury and less efficient at repairing the problem.

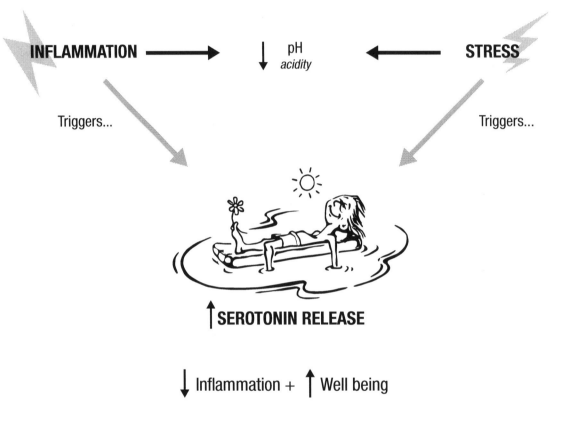

INFLAMMATION → ↓ pH *acidity* ← **STRESS**

Triggers...   Triggers...

↑ **SEROTONIN RELEASE**

↓ Inflammation + ↑ Well being

DIAGRAM 3.2A (I) HOW WE COPE WITH BOTH INFLAMMATION AND STRESS: RELEASE FEEL-GOOD SEROTONIN: Serotonin gives us control of inflammation and a sense of well being. For this reason both inflammatory episodes and stress cause the release of serotonin.

**CHRONIC/PROLONGED
INFLAMMATION &/OR STRESS**

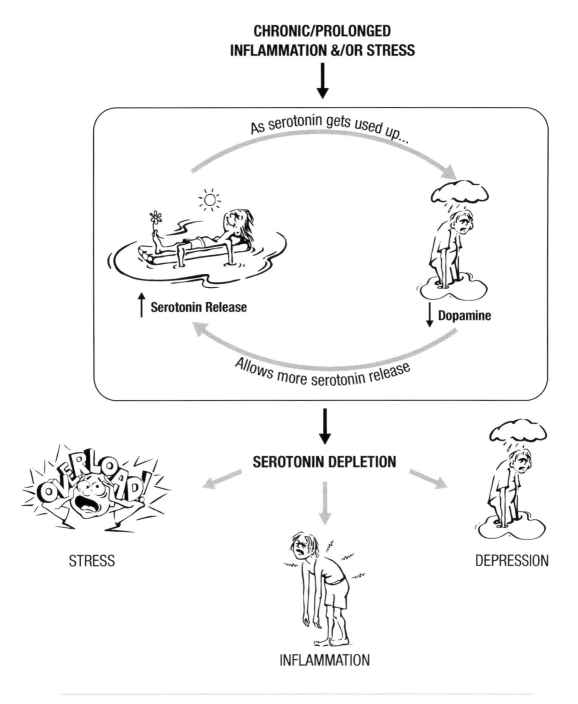

DIAGRAM 3.2A (II) ENDLESS LOOP OF INFLAMMATION RELATED TO SEROTONIN DEPLETION: Prolonged inflammation and stress can cause an endless loop of serotonin depletion that results in depression and *more* inflammation.

Generally, when stress is a significant factor in someone's pain, I find it usually is a level of stress suddenly out of the ordinary for that person, but many people, without realizing it, have come to live in a heightened state of stress on a daily basis. While these chronically stressed people may be managing it well enough not to let it show, that stress might be simmering in a way that is pushing the body pH to a tipping point. With this kind of constant influx of inflammatory stress chemicals into the body, it doesn't have to take much of any other kind of inflammation trigger to suddenly develop a case of everyday pain in some seemingly random body part.

Now back to the matter of stress addiction. This is where things get interesting: Some of the key molecules involved with the response to inflammation ("mediators of inflammation") also moonlight as, and communicate closely with, *mood-altering* chemicals in the brain and nervous system!

Serotonin is one of the most important mediators of inflammation. Not only does it help with vasodilation (allowing more helper molecules to the site of injury for clean-up), it is the one mediator that also keeps the inflammatory response from getting out of control by limiting the release of one of the other mediators,[viii] thereby keeping a check on what could become an out-of-control snowball effect. Serotonin is *also* that chemical in the brain and body that we hear so much about because it plays a key role in helping to regulate sleep, body temperature, libido and appetite (Diagram 3.2A (i)). When it's not present in adequate quantities, it has been associated with depression.

Here's the hitch: When we are stressed, we unwittingly force the production and release of serotonin through a complex series of events. And why not, if it helps us feel better and keeps a lid on the destructive stress hormones?[ix] Unfortunately, a *high and sustained* concentration of serotonin in the body is found to deplete dopamine—a key player in mood regulation.

Serotonin goes up. Dopamine goes down.

Decreased dopamine levels have been associated with major depression.[x] More depression signals the need for more feel-good, anti-inflammatory serotonin and, if the effects of stress are left unchecked, eventually we also become serotonin *depleted*. Symptoms of serotonin depletion include an increase in carbohydrate cravings (sugars, breads, alcohol). Guess what? These carbs *do* indeed help: they trigger serotonin release from our reserves, which gives us a brief hit of "ahhhh…," *but*, unfortunately, they also decrease body pH, which we now know causes inflammation (Diagram 3.2A (ii)).

If we've become serotonin depleted (from a sustained chronic state of stress), there is no longer any straightforward way to decrease this simmering inflammation—the unwitting product of stress itself. Any kind of simmering inflammation is a perfect recipe for a case of full-blown inflammation popping up at the drop of a hat, but especially now that we've lost our main "keep inflammation in check" molecule—serotonin; we've used it all up. That's problem number one.

The larger and more complex problem—number two—is the decrease in dopamine levels that all of this serotonin overproduction—and now depletion—has triggered. The body is marvelously adaptive and will do its best to fix this imbalance by doing what it can to increase dopamine levels.

So, how does it do this….?

Well, Here's How:

Depression is not considered an acceptable road to survival from the perspective of our reptilian brain. It does not fit into any of our predetermined blueprints for optimal functioning. If you don't have the get-up-and-go to get out from under the covers or to care for yourself, there's probably less chance that you'll be feeling foxy enough to try finding a mate or have the spunk to effectively outrun large predators. Having made this assessment, the body makes an ingenious attempt to increase our chance for "survival" by kicking on the next best mechanism, which happens to be the system that releases endorphins—the fight-or-flight response.[10] Suddenly, rather than being chemically depressed (i.e., dopamine deficient), we find ourselves coping with the day-to-day grind by cranking out oodles of adrenaline left and right, often via inconvenient and badly timed spurts.

---

10. The fight-or-flight response is the reaction that all animals have to acute, life-threatening stress. If someone or something is about to attack you, your body goes into survival mode and you may either run like you never knew you could run or you get ready to beat off the attacker. Both choices become possible because of a sudden biologic discharge of chemicals that cause a chain reaction that allows us a short burst of extraordinary strength, resilience and blood flow to all the necessary systems of the body.

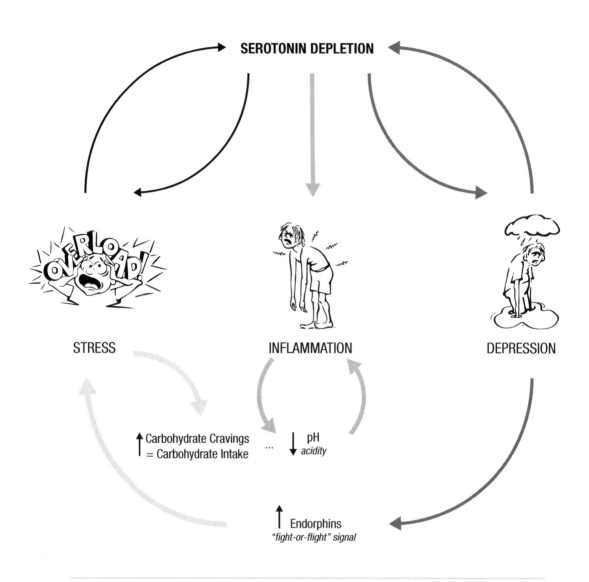

SEROTONIN DEPLETION

STRESS

INFLAMMATION

DEPRESSION

↑ Carbohydrate Cravings = Carbohydrate Intake

... ↓ pH *acidity*

↑ Endorphins *"fight-or-flight" signal*

DIAGRAM 3.2B THE VICIOUS CYCLE BETWEEN INFLAMMATION, STRESS AND DEPRESSION: Each imbalance can perpetuate the other. Stress prolongs recovery from injury. Prolonged inflammation and pain feed the need to release stress hormones. Chronic stress leads to depression. Depression can lead to endorphin/adrenalin release and carbohydrate cravings. Carbohydrates cause a drop in pH (increased acidity). Tissue acidity predisposes the body to inflammation. Meanwhile, endorphins are keeping the stress level high, and it goes on.

Conveniently, however, this is exactly what raises our dopamine levels. Success! (Or is it…?) Dopamine is another feel-good chemical. When levels are low, major depression can result. When levels spike suddenly, we get what amounts to a bucket of ice water in the face. Dopamine has been linked to motivation, optimism and pleasure[xi] as well as reward (although that latter idea is not without controversy).[xii] This increase in feel-good dopamine rewards our brain for being in a constant state of stress. So, even if that means periodic panic attacks, lack of sleep, or poor digestion, all of these things are regarded as lesser side effects in exchange for what is a more important survival alternative: get up and go. Being in a constant state of stress continues to assure that we stay in a depleted serotonin state. Stress hormone precursors to adrenaline have direct effects on inflammation in the body.[xiii,xiv] In other words, stress hormones increase potential for and can *cause* inflammation (Diagram 3.2B).

When all other systems are functioning optimally, flooding the body with stress-related chemical soup may not in itself result in pain. But should we happen to add to this delicate balance, an innocent physical trauma—large or small—sets the stage for a longer, much more puzzling road back to being pain free.

Stress IS all in your head…and everywhere else.

Let's go back to **BILLIE'S** story for a moment: what was it exactly that she was intending to come see me for before her neck froze up on her so vigorously? You might recall that Billie meant to schedule an appointment with me for something that she wasn't even sure I could help her with, but when her neck froze up unexpectedly that's what got her in the office. The symptoms she was having before that time began about four months ago and seemed to always be triggered by some sort of arm motion or position of the arms—she demonstrates by raising her arm outstretched in front of her—or even at times just when gesturing with her arms and hands while speaking.

> "Some of the key molecules involved with the response to inflammation also moonlight as mood-altering chemicals in the brain and nervous system."

What seems to happen is that she experiences a sudden sensation of numbness and tingling from the back of her upper arms down into the whole arm and hand. One time she was reaching into the fridge and had something in her hand that she dropped because of one of these episodes, which led her to realize that there is also a feeling of weakness that lingers even after resuming neutral arm position at her sides. She'll also suddenly feel an increase in her heart rate and a feeling of chest pressure that seems to make breathing difficult. And, at times, she develops sudden headache in conjunction with all of this, which then lasts for the rest of the day. There have been seven of these incidents within the last four months, and this is a completely new experience for her.

Billie's symptoms sound like they could be due to some scary neurologic or cardiovascular event or defect, but before coming to see me she checked with all the right doctors who performed the appropriate tests and asked all the right questions. All investigations came up with no sign of any outright disease process—other than some borderline high blood pressure that she was already aware of. While this is good news, it still leaves her with a perplexing and uncomfortable problem.

More delving into her background reveals that Billie is most definitely at her wits' end with work stress. She is very good at it but does not enjoy her job. She enjoys the people, but, by the same token, this leaves her unable to say no to the many demands being put on her. She recognizes she is doing far too much and putting in far too many hours. Her personal time, her sleep and her energy and mental health are all being compromised. She feels she is just surviving day to day and barely at that. The onset of these very unsettling symptoms has shown her that there are real consequences to the stress she is under and she has resolved to begin to do something about it—starting with bodywork treatments.

It's true that maybe Billie has some cardiovascular risk factors. She may have some weight that could stand to be transformed into muscle. She may not always make the right food choices, but each one of these things alone would not necessarily be causing her physical discomfort. For Billie, the work stress is a much bigger influence on her physical health than she was realizing; she is starting to see her bucket overflowing because of it.

Hopefully by now it's becoming more apparent to you that controlling stress is an important part of controlling and resolving pain, and not just because stress can cause us to tighten up our muscles. If the pain and inflammation of chemical imbalance is as intertwined with stress hormones as the literature implies, then we really can't help but consider the influence of other emotional experiences—not just stress.

CHAPTER 4

Emotional Triggers

WHILE THE IMPACTS OF PHYSICAL OR chemical imbalance on pain are tangible concepts, how emotional strain can contribute to the experience of pain is a much less concrete idea and not as easy to grasp. Yet this is something we all have experienced on a physical level at some point in our lives. Who hasn't felt a loss of appetite in times of grief or extreme elation? Or, how about moments of embarrassment as an awkward teenager—a sudden facial flush or a case of sweaty palms? Then there's the very common phenomenon of feeling your heart race during an unexpected fright or a happy excitement.

The emotional brain and body should not be taken lightly when pain is concerned. The phrase and attitude, "It's all in your head," meaning, "It doesn't really exist," is completely outdated. It turns out that it *is* all in our heads and thereby within all the tissues of our body! We now know that there is a direct relationship between some of the chemicals involved with emotional stress and the pain-causing chemicals of inflammation. Some of the medications that pharmaceutical manufacturers are promoting for chronic pain are actually just new uses of existing medications that have been used to treat depression and anxiety for decades. These new uses are in large part rooted in the knowledge and evidence that now exists about brain chemistry's effect on inflammation in the body.

We have something called *neuropeptide receptors* in all of our tissues and structures. Psychopharmacologist Candace Pert, PhD, describes neuropeptide receptors as "locations all over the body where information converges."[xv] Neuropeptides are signaling molecules released by parts of our nervous system and the neuropeptide *receptors* are communication hubs. The neuropeptide signals or messages are received for interpretation and implementation at these receptor sites in places like muscles, blood vessels and glands—where specific cells can be told to either spring into action or lie low. An example of a commonly known neuropeptide signal is epinephrine, also referred to as adrenaline. So, for instance, when adrenaline is released we might feel some muscles tighten or we might feel suddenly cold, hot, sweaty or dry-mouthed.

The release of neuropeptides like this can be initiated or affected by our emotions. It takes some practice, but we all are capable of controlling our emotions to some degree given the chance to learn how. Meditation is one example of how to change the body's neuropeptide signaling by taking control of our state of mind. Not only does our state of mind affect how we perceive pain, but it also affects the very chemistry of the body that governs chemical causes of pain.

Posture—Chicken or Egg?

The idea of this connection between body chemistry, emotions and the pain of inflammation is certainly fascinating and could lead to endless discussion, but no matter what, it's our state of mind—both conscious and unconscious—that plays a huge role in determining postural tendencies. In other words, how we hold and maneuver our bodies while upright and moving against gravity is in large part controlled by how we *feel* about ourselves and our world.

As we discussed earlier in the section on mechanical triggers, postural tendencies definitely predispose us to areas of structural weakness and pain. There's no disputing that state of mind and mood can be linked with how we physically hold ourselves. "Each emotion is experienced throughout the organism and not in just the head or body," says Dr. Pert, who summarized ideas put forth by Paul Ekman, PhD, a psychologist and behavioral scientist who has extensively researched body language, facial expression and how it correlates with emotion. How often can you look at someone and immediately know their mood? Another revealing perspective on how the body expresses emotion is explored in the book *Emotional Anatomy* by Stanley Keleman.[xvi] In it are presented visual and structural investigations of deflated (depressive) postures, inflated (elated) postures and several degrees in between (Figure 4.1).

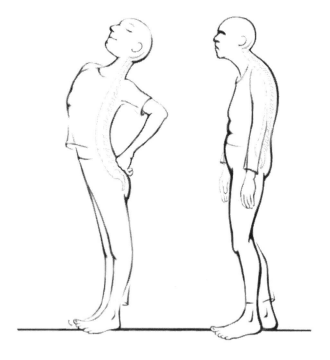

FIGURE 4.1 POSTURE AND MOOD: How you feel about yourself and your place in the world affects your posture, which affects your potential for pain due to the resulting structural imbalance unique to how you carry your emotions.

Take this concept a step further, and it becomes clear that our very sense of self and how we see our place in the world and in relationship to others influences our posture as well. Subtle attitudes like these have real ramifications on our pain because of the way those feelings are displayed through aspects of our daily body language. Body positioning and habitual posturing is a very big part of what can either render us vulnerable to physical strain or be used by us with intention to increase our resilience against physical strain. Let's look at how this plays out in Charlene's case.

The "me" you see vs. the "me" I feel

As a dancer, **CHARLENE** can attest to the immense pressure in the performance community to adhere to (admittedly antiquated) standards for body presentation. To some degree in the modern dance culture, there is less demand for waif-like bodies and natural curves are definitely embraced, but many of the dancers have some background in ballet, where there has always been an undercurrent of this notion that pelvic tuck is paramount. My dancer patients struggle with this when I explain my objections to them about it and the mechanical strain it causes. It challenges some long-held beliefs about the basics of dance, but this obsession with pelvic tucking is not unique to the dance world. The idea that we should tuck our buttocks in and suck the gut in seems to permeate all corners of society. The good intention behind this pelvic-tuck culture is to engage the "core" in order to protect the spine, but, in fact, the focus on tucking is doing quite the opposite for most of us. Engaging the core is much more than simply tucking and sucking things in. There is no structural strength or power in a tucked pelvis and a flattened spine (Figure 4.2).

Good intentions are one thing, but body image is another big factor in the tuck phenomenon. I think many of us at some point in our lives begin to feel self conscious about those parts of our bodies (the butt and the belly) and we decide that it is somehow more polite to keep that rear end from sticking out and under no circumstances should anyone see that you have a belly—the same belly that everyone else is trying to hide, too. This creates a situation for the spine that is exactly the opposite of what we need for balance and strength.

Flattening the lower back is not good for you—plain and simple. When you lie on the floor there should be a natural little hollow under your lower back. If there isn't, then you can bet that your upper back and neck are doing more work than they should when your body is in the upright position. When posture is linked with beliefs about body image like this—we often aren't aware of it.

After her pregnancy, Charlene was filled with self-imposed pressure to not only lose the baby weight but also to return to dance and yoga while embodying the stereotypical images associated with these disciplines that she strived to portray for years. Combine this image of what she learned—the correct way to hold her body during performance, and this false idea of what good posture is (tuck it in—suck it in), together with a self-consciousness of the extra baby belly—and it all took its toll. The amount of time she spent holding "it" in is what caused her sensation of leg tightness by creating friction and irritation on nerves in the back that would normally be protected and comfortably housed in a spine with a nice, gentle lower back arch (buttocks *out*, belly *out* and relaxed). Eventually this is what made her already hardworking mid-back give way that day, when it felt to her as though all she was doing was walking. Think about what a serious shift in self-image it takes to allow the body to go from rigid and tucked to loose and bulbous.

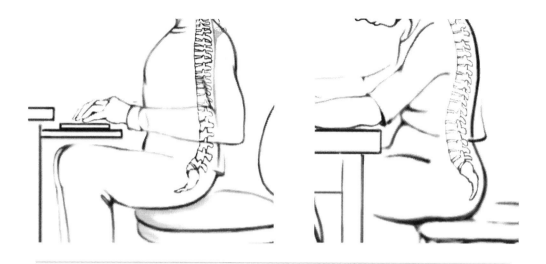

FIGURE 4.2 SITTING WITH PELVIS TUCKED VS. SITTING WELL:
Tucking the belly causes lower back stress in the spine. This creates conflict between the back muscles and the front muscles. Letting the buttocks stick out and letting the belly relax allows the spine to take its natural shape, which maintains peaceful balance.

One of the most challenging aspects of treatment that I see with my patients is the shift in *attitude* that needs to take place before any advice on posture can really be embodied and incorporated on a daily basis in a way that leads to *lasting* relief from repetitive mechanical strain. This shift has to be about our sense of how we physically occupy space and, ironically, in all of the non-physical aspects. This change in attitude is often the final piece in the puzzle to resolving everyday pain. After all other mechanical and chemical influences have been sufficiently tamed, there are these subtleties about how we present ourselves in the world that need re-working. This last piece of treatment is about how we hold ourselves—head, hips and shoulders—when relating to others, when gesturing at our phones, when entranced by our computer screens or sitting in a meeting deflecting tensions. All of these physical expressions rest within each of us at a deep emotional level and can't truly be taught or untaught in a passive way. In other words, nobody can do it for us. It's up to each of us to seek out and implement. With the help of a trained eye, though, we can become aware of some of these postural habits. Only with this awareness, and combined with some dogged

> "Not only
> does our
> state of mind
> affect how we
> perceive pain,
> but it also
> affects the
> very chemistry
> of the body
> that governs
> pain."

determination, can we experience positive and lasting shifts toward avoiding everyday pain. As we take repeated action to adjust how the body supports itself in all situations, we make possible for ourselves a sense of greater ease.[11]

As it turns out, we have come full circle in our discussion of the triggers of pain and inflammation; we've come back to looking at *mechanical* imbalance as a source of pain, albeit due in some cases to emotions. Hopefully at this point you have a better perspective on how the body's mechanical imbalance can be influenced by and co-exists with chemical and emotional factors. With a wide–angle perspective it appears that no lone factor (physical, chemical or emotional) can or should ever be singled out without consideration of the other two. It's something that alternative and not-so-alternative health care approaches have recognized for centuries. It's really what *should* be implied by the modern idea of "wholistic" health care, but as individuals—patients and doctors alike—it is our nature to focus on the hope for a single quick fix. We get lost in believing what mainstream marketers would have us think—that pain is the direct result of either one thing *or* another—not in fact a complex balancing act between all three aspects—mechanical, chemical *and* emotional—which can certainly be an overwhelming notion.

True health comes from finding our individual balance between all three of these influences in our everyday life. Finding this balance is not quick nor easy, and for some of us not always as instinctual as we would like, even though we all clearly have the potential to be our own best detectives in health. It's true that this balancing

---

11. Examples of areas of bodywork that can facilitate this sort of relearning and repatterning include the Alexander technique and the Feldenkrais method.

act is constantly in flux, but it is something we are all capable of achieving and maintaining with the right information and guidance. Hopefully, with the help of this book as your guide, you will find that perhaps you only needed a little reminder of what your body has already known about how to be free from everyday pain.

A Word About Genes, Epigenetics and Genomics

Our genetic code is a very important part of what's at the root of why none of us respond identically to the same stressors and, for that reason, deserves at least an honorable mention. The science of epigenetics and genomics is relatively young and we have yet to fully understand what influences expression of our genes' potential. One example of the role that genes play in inflammation is in regard to the acid-base balance of the body. Our pH levels are largely at the mercy of our body's enzyme response to the presence of waste and toxins. The types and quantities of helpful enzymes we come equipped with are dictated by our genes[xvii] to a large degree. There's no clearer way to explain the pointlessness in comparing ourselves to others when pain is concerned. We all have the potential for optimal health with minimal inflammation. We all just have very different thresholds to surmount to get ourselves there, *but* the principles presented in Section I of this book are the same across the board. These differences in our genetic make-up are why some of us will have to rely more heavily on the exercise portion of the equation and others may have to rely more heavily on the nutrient balance while still others may find that stress management is the key to finding *their* optimal balance.

SUMMARY:
Section I — Why Does it Hurt?

Pain = Inflammation

BUT...

Inflammation doesn't always = Pain...right away

Triggers can push inflammation over the edge and *then* lead to pain:

MECHANICAL TRIGGERS:

- ✓ Compression
- ✓ Lengthening
- ✓ Shearing

CHEMICAL TRIGGERS:

- ✓ pH Imbalance (low pH (acidic) leads to inflammation)
- ✓ Injured Tissue and Repair Molecules
- ✓ Waste Back-Up
- ✓ Stress Chemicals

EMOTIONAL TRIGGERS:

- ✓ Stress Contributes to Chemical Triggers
- ✓ Self-Image Contributes to Mechanical Triggers

Section II:

How Do I Make it Stop?

CHAPTER 5

Cool the Fire: Address Those Mechanical Triggers

DO YOU REMEMBER WHEN YOU WERE a kid and you learned what to do if you were to catch on fire? Well, you have pain because your body is essentially on fire from inflammation, so, if you're going to put a stop to it, the sensible thing to do would be to approach pain exactly the same way:

Stop, Drop and Roll!

Well, okay, maybe not *exactly* the same way you would in order to put out actual flames, but let's take a closer look at what we *can* do with that darned fire of inflammation.

"It's so important to respect the pain right away."

Stop!

First and foremost, it's essential to immediately stop fanning the flames.

If someone actually catches on fire, the act of stopping in your tracks will keep the flow of air around the body from feeding the flames. The more you run around, the more air the flames get—which makes them burn harder and faster. When dealing with the fire of inflammation related to sudden pain of the everyday variety (not from serious or chronic disease), if we don't stop in our tracks immediately we also risk feeding those flames. Many of us are constantly doing things with and to our bodies that, without even realizing it, easily feed the fire of inflammation—just like running around would feed flames if we were actually burning.

Most of the time, when the body is not in an injured or weakened condition, all those inflammatory behaviors or situations don't actually cause any pain. So it's no wonder we have no idea how problematic some of these situations can be until there is noticeable discomfort. When there *is* finally pain, it just means we suddenly lost our usually generous buffer for dealing with minor imperfections in movement, positioning or body chemistry.

The tissues of the body, when compromised and in pain, are too inflamed already to accommodate any additional, inadvertent inflammation that can come from any number of familiar daily behaviors or positions. It makes sense that your body would have a shorter fuse before bursting into flames if it's being asked to do more work while already overwhelmed.

Drop!

Really? To the floor? Yes, literally to the floor—both for real flames and when everyday pain strikes. Again, if you're actually on fire, dropping to the floor is the next step in taking away the main thing that keeps fire burning: air.

The best way to make a lot of everyday pain stop is to take the most volatile fuel out of the equation: the compressive stress of gravity. Compression is one of three main mechanical irritants that can ignite or sustain the fire of inflammation.[12] In an emergency it's best to just give in to it. Lie down.

Now, sometimes *how* you lie down makes all the difference. Here we'll have to recall some of the ideas introduced in Chapter 1 about the blueprint for optimal mechanical balance. What you'll see as you read on is that there is a combination of "passive release" positioning techniques that are very effective at restoring neutral spine positioning, with very low impact. Sometimes when these positioning techniques are implemented early on, these alone can restore the necessary balance to the skeleton and resolve the pain. Restoring structural harmony among your bones will signal to the distressed and therefore pain-causing soft tissues to disengage and cool off.

Roll!

Rolling back and forth on the ground is what you're supposed to do to put out the flames with finality and make sure they don't reignite. All that is left after you roll is the damage the flames left behind—hopefully only to the superficial layers of fabric, if you acted quickly enough.

Once you've stopped and dropped and done some passive release work on the floor for your pain, it also eventually becomes time to *roll*. No, don't try to roll back and forth like you would if you were really on fire. But, when you're feeling injured, make sure you do always take the time and extra effort to roll to your side before you try to get up. Because your tissues are now "damaged" by the fire, they won't perform the way you're used to, so this will be your best way to make sure the inflammation doesn't reignite with a vengeance right away. Rolling to your side before getting up off the floor, bed or treatment table is going to be an important modification that will allow repair to happen as quickly as possible.

No matter where the pain is—neck, mid-back or low back—how we get up from lying down is one of *the* most important things to pay attention to when we're

---

12. The other two are lengthening and shearing forces, as we saw in Chapter 2.

in pain. If we ignore and try to power through this potentially aggravating transition, we will significantly slow down our recovery and take several steps back in our progress each and every time we get up out of bed or off the floor. The importance of this will hopefully become clear to you as you read on.

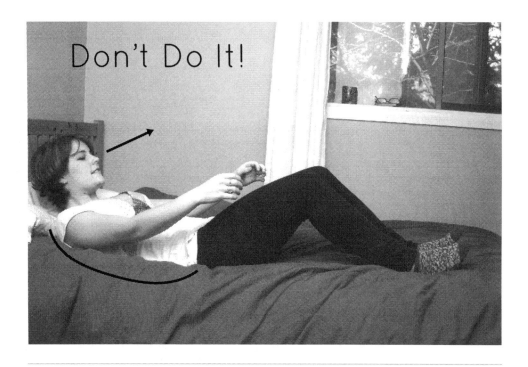

PHOTO 5.1: Sitting up like this to get up either out of bed, off the couch, off the floor or off a massage table will stress your spine and can set the stage for injury whether or not it feels that way to you.

Photo 5.1 depicts what is one of the biggest problems with what patients with everyday pain do when they go home from receiving even the best and most helpful treatment in the world—no matter what modality that might have been. All it takes is something like this sort of really common activity to undo all of the good that therapy might have done. *And,* it's not anything that anyone suspects would be a problem at all because it's something everyone does for most of their lives. The people who *do* understand this are the ones who have had *really* bad episodes of back pain that leave no other option.

Once you have implemented the stop, drop and roll technique, you've success-fully shown yourself that you *can* put out the fire; it's within your control, even if only temporarily. Now is also the time to see what you can do about recruiting early intervention. Get help! Pick a style of bodywork that you like and that's easily acces-sible to you—making it easy is key. The path of least resistance is worth a million bucks when you're in pain. Whatever sounds good to you is what you should do. What you *shouldn't* do is nothing.

It's really important to get an outside perspective on what's happening with your body. Someone who deals with analyzing structure and function on a daily basis will be able to give your body guidance that can really speed up your recovery. Then, based on what you learn from that input, you can more effectively complement the bodywork or acupuncture with some of this early-stage home care (stopping, dropping and rolling) or some of the other modifications to your daily routine that you will have help figuring out in Section III.

It's so important to respect the pain right away: figure out what it's telling you. You have to use that information to do what you can in order to avoid being in pain again in the future. Start yourself down the right path as quickly as possible by stopping, restoring balance and reducing stress and you may not even have to bother too much with trying to figure out what the pain is telling you. But that only works if you act right away.

The problem with putting off taking care of our pain is that the longer we allow pain to exist, the more entrenched it can become. Think of the pain of inflammation like a corrosive substance such as bleach or acid. Suppose we were to spill one of those things onto our clothes, for example. If it sits undisturbed, it will slowly erode the integrity of the clothing and eventually you'll see a hole. The hole can still be patched, but it will never be the same and there will always be a noticeable reminder of the damage caused. If you take early measures and rinse the bleach or acid off right away, the damage will be minimal and you may never have to think about it again (until there is more wear and tear in the same area, maybe years later).

By living with pain no matter how minor it is, what we are actually doing is teaching our body—the nervous system, our biochemical regulators and our struc-ture—how to *be* in pain, how to successfully coexist with the pain. Too many of us have come to see this (living with some amount of pain) as a badge of honor, but the pain—just like bleach or acid—will wear away at us and our nervous system and can leave permanent damage even after the fire has been put out.

The body in its true brilliance will learn to accommodate the pain and can develop habits and mechanisms in response to it so that we are still either able to function with the pain in the background or function at a lower level to avoid it. These initially smart adaptations can come back to bite us years down the road when we finally pile on maybe just one too many stressors to the already precarious balance. More importantly, however, allowing pain to reside unchallenged allows it to become the path of least resistance by sensitizing our pain-detecting nerve endings.[xviii] This means the ability of those nerves to feel pain slowly switches to overdrive. So, even though you can get good at mentally blocking it out, you're actually physiologically or biologically allowing your nerves to *learn* how to be in pain and how to signal pain with increasing ease.

If you're having pain, remember that pain equals inflammation even if you can't see the heat, redness or swelling. Let's figure out how to put out that hot fire of inflam-mation at the root of your acute or early-stage pain. As we learned in Chapter 1, all inflammatory triggers can be broken down into these three categories: mechanical, biochemical and emotional. The mechanical triggers are often the easiest to modify for immediate results, so you'll find that much of this chapter on how to make the pain stop at its initial onset is about addressing the mechanical trigger first.

Cooling the Fire: Start by Stopping

Do you remember from Chapter 1 the idea of comparing two people walking on a treadmill at identical speeds and lengths of time as an illustration of how inflammatory thresholds can vary? The treadmill served as the inflammatory trigger in this example. Using this same image, consider the fact that, if you are going to put a stop to the inflammation, then you have to cool the fire by getting off that treadmill (Figure 5.1). You simply have to put a stop to it.

Get Off the Treadmill!

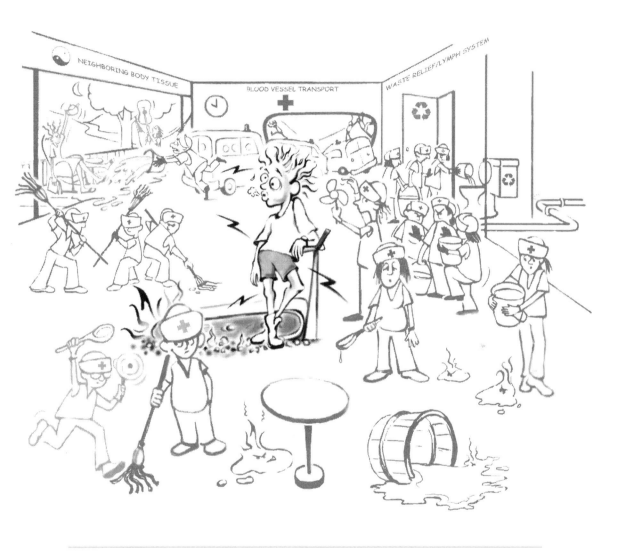

FIGURE 5.1 STOP—ELIMINATE ALL THE STRESS TRIGGERS OF PAIN: Get off the treadmill to give your body a chance to deal with the mess.

Stop all the things that are stressing your structure and the mechanical function of this structure. You feel pain? Maybe you feel just a "tweak"? Stop yourself in your tracks before it gets worse. Before the pain can stop, *you* have to stop. Eliminate the stressors—those inflammation triggers. Recall from Chapter 2 that the three main mechanical stressors are:

1. Compression
2. Lengthening
3. Shearing forces

Let's look at how to address these one at a time starting with Figure 5.2.

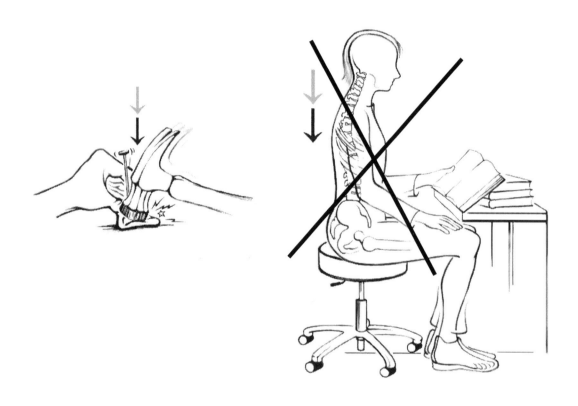

FIGURE 5.2 STOP SITTING AND STANDING—ELIMINATE THE COMPRESSIVE STRESS: The first step in stopping a flare-up of everyday pain is to eliminate the compressive stress of gravity—the most volatile fuel of the fire.

Stop the Compression!

How do we stop compression? Lie down! As soon as you can—just lay your body down. Forget trying to look cool. Forget trying to power forward. It's just not worth it.

As I mentioned at the beginning of this chapter, though, *how* you lie down makes all the difference. Your immediate goal should be to reduce mechanical triggers. This means helping the spine find its natural neutral shape with the least amount of pressure on it. Once you're on the ground and on your back, if there's still pain, don't panic right away. First, try to implement this all-purpose, go-to spine neutralizing relief-positioning shown in Photo 5.2.

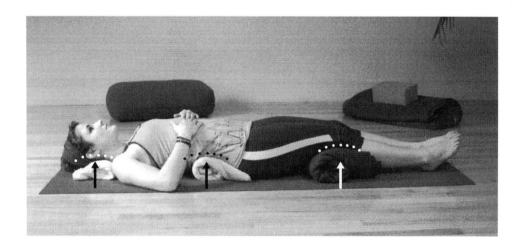

PHOTO 5.2 SPINE-NEUTRALIZING RELIEF POSITIONING: To neutralize the stress on your spine, lie down with these three points supported. One towel goes under the neck. The rolled-up diameter of the neck towel should be approximately the size of your palm. One towel goes under the small of your back. The rolled-up diameter of the lower back towel should also be the diameter of your palm. Place a third, larger roll–towel or pillow under the knees. The key is to rest all of your muscles and allow the towels to push your spine back to neutral. You will feel your body adjusting to the change. This may feel like an uncomfortable stretch. Stay like this until the sensation lessens. Make sure to roll to your side to get in and out of this position! If this increases pain, of course stop and seek help.

Without fail, this passive release will maximally neutralize the spine and remove any undue pressure. Sometimes if there is a lot of inflammation, this position can initially feel uncomfortable. But, rest assured, because this positioning is promoting what we know to be an optimal shape for the spinal column and in the least stressful position possible, the discomfort you feel here is generally safe to relax into. If there is discomfort, it is just from inflammation itself and the body's unfamiliarity with this position, but it is not doing any damage. This is the kind of "productive" discomfort that sometimes happens when we "walk backward" through an injury with corrective bodywork or positioning release work during the early stages of a strain. If you've ever dislocated a shoulder severely enough that it needed to be manually relocated, then you know the pain of going backward through an injury. This is an extreme example, but once it's back in that socket it feels well worth it!

You might be thinking that, when you're in pain, getting in and out of this position doesn't sound like much fun and you're right. The process of hoisting yourself up and down or in and out of these restorative release positions can easily destroy any of the benefit—that is, if you don't approach it with a safe plan of attack. Rolling to your side is going to be your best bet and from this day forward will probably be a technique you should use any time you need to maneuver yourself up from lying down—even when you are not in pain.

The Safe Way to Get Up—Part 1

Bend Your Knees:

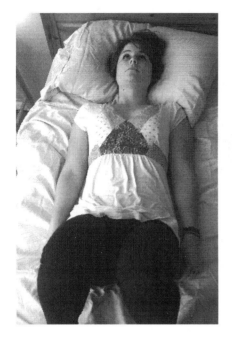

Feet hip width apart

Press down with feet and tighten buttocks

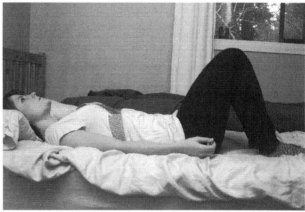

Lift Pelvis and Shift Sideways:

Keep buttocks tight for protection

Push into your feet

Move your hips away from the edge of the bed

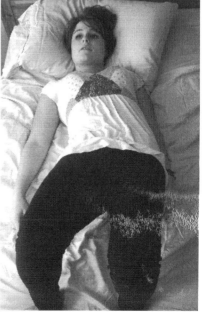

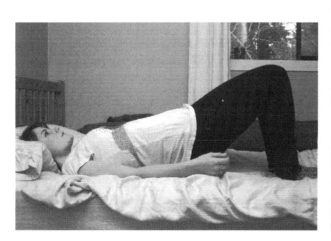

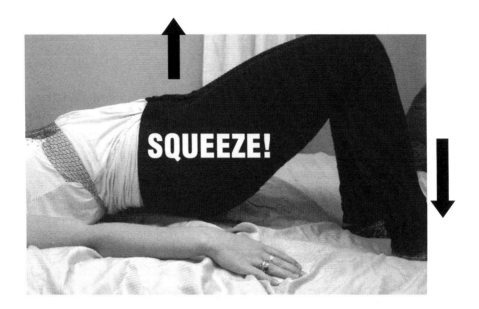

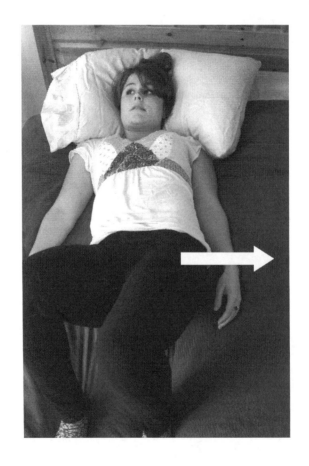

The Safe Way to Get Up – Part 2

Arm Push/Leg Counterbalance:

Push with elbow and hand into mattress

At the same time: Let legs and feet fall off the edge of bed

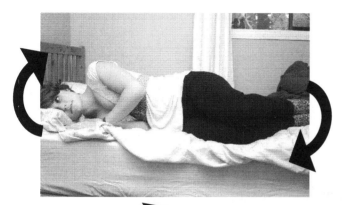

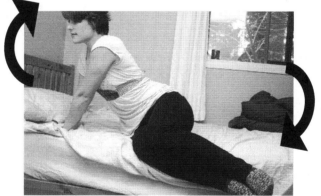

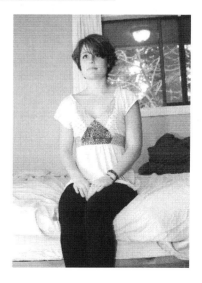

Always Remember:

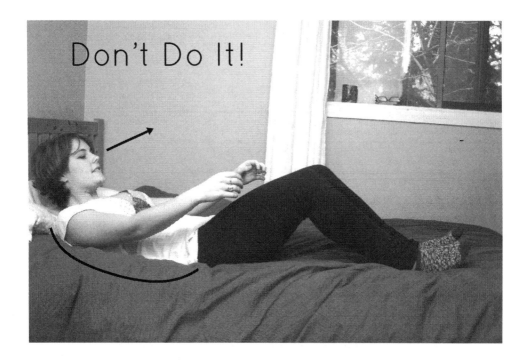

So you may *think* you have a strong "core" because you've always paid attention to your abdominal workouts and, if you've worked so hard to have strong abs, you should be able to do a simple sit-up to get out of bed—right? Wrong.

It is, in my opinion, *never* a good idea to sit straight up after you've been resting on your back—no matter how strong you are and how resilient you feel. You'll just be pushing your luck and flirting with disaster somewhere along the road.

For someone who's in pain, sitting up this way is not just a bad idea, but sometimes it's just plain impossible.[xix] I'm not just talking about lower back pain, either. This applies to neck and mid-back pain as well.

First of all, it should be pointed out that the term "core" is often misinterpreted and mistakenly used when referring to "abdominal muscles" and vice versa. Abdominal muscles are strictly superficial—covering the contents of the abdomen, whereas the "core" should be acknowledged to include the muscles directly around the spine—deep underneath the intestines, inside of the pelvis as well as some of the deep *back* muscles. This setup is not unlike an apple with its fleshy meat: peel on the outside and core at the very center. The apple peel and some of the outer flesh is to the apple core what the abdominal muscles are to our spinal core.

These deep core muscles far away from the surface are the "primary spinal stabilizers." They are the muscles that are busy holding your vertebrae up on top of each other, preventing collapse and compression all day long. You can do crunches and sit ups until you're blue in the face and you may not be using even one of these core muscles at all. In fact, you risk injuring your back by doing traditional abdominal strengthening in the gym without first giving due diligence to your *actual* core and back muscles (Figure 5.3).

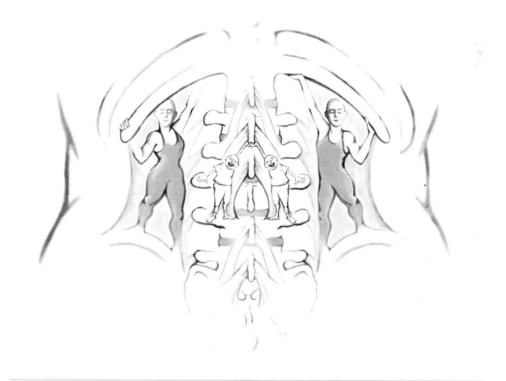

FIGURE 5.3 TRUE CORE MUSCLES—THE SPINAL STABILIZERS: These stabilizers are deep inside the body. The ones right against the spinal bones are collectively called the "multifidi." The multifidus muscles are small but charged with the big job of holding up the vertebral bones and preventing collapse all day long. The larger, more powerful muscles farther away from the spine are better at providing limited bursts of motion and effort.

It's been shown that the primary stabilizers of the spine (the true, deep core muscles) actually turn *off* (become unavailable to us) in the presence of a strain because of something called *reflex inhibition.*[xx,xxi] The muscles that support the spine become inhibited, and they just stop working when there's pain or risk of further injury. Often there's pain *because* these support muscles (usually the multifidi) stopped working. But, it's a feedback loop and because these two things—pain and muscle inhibition—enable and reinforce each other, when you have one (pain), you definitely have the other (muscle inhibition; Figure 5.4).

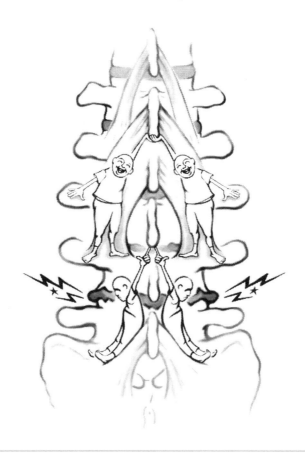

FIGURE 5.4 REFLEX INHIBITION—WHEN THE MULTIFIDI (STABI-LIZERS) TURN OFF AND PAIN STARTS: "Reflex inhibition" is the protective response to strain or sprain at the level of the spinal joint. The role of this protective response turns *off* the multifidi to protect from overstretch/tearing. Unfortunately, this leaves little protection from compression at the intervertebral joint and essentially puts the disk under greater stress.

Another complication to this phenomenon is that sometimes "strain"—the very thing that can set this whole dysfunctional loop in motion (as it's perceived by the body's reflex inhibition mechanism)— can be something simple and sneaky like just being *inactive* for an extended period of time—for example, sitting in a rounded, slouched position[xxii] (Figure 5.5).

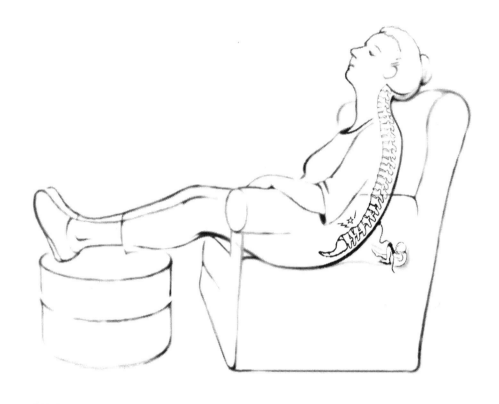

FIGURE 5.5 A COMMON TRIGGER OF REFLEX INHIBITION: This very common position when prolonged causes reflex inhibition, disabling our spinal stabilizers and putting our larger back muscles in the position of having to take over.

When the small (but essential) muscles of the spine don't work because they've inconveniently turned themselves off, the big muscles have to take over and do their best to fight the fight of keeping things from getting worse, *but*, in doing so, can actually do more harm than good. Figure 5.6 illustrates why it is such a struggle for these larger muscle groups to do the work of the little guys.

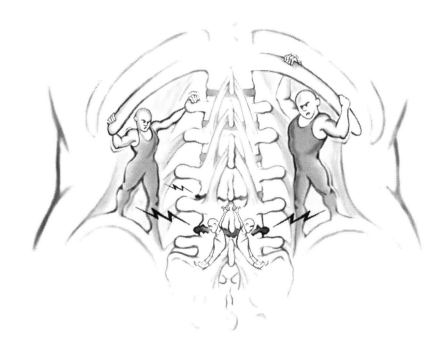

FIGURE 5.6 COMPENSATION FOR REFLEX INHIBITION BY LARGE MOVER MUSCLES: When the primary spinal stabilizers become disabled, we depend on the larger surrounding muscles to take over. These larger muscles are capable of strong bursts of activity but are not designed to do the steady work of the stabilizers, so we experience not only pain and tightness but also exhaustion when this happens.

When we have back or neck pain, it's very often because of reflex inhibition gone wrong. Deep spinal muscles and ligaments sensing excessive stretch are programmed to yield to that stretch in order to avoid further injury that could result from fighting the pull. Unfortunately, when these overstretched muscles and ligaments let go to protect themselves from injury, we are left without any of the deep spinal stability that they usually provide. Instead, we start to feel pain and tension in the larger superficial muscle groups trying too hard to do a job they were not intended for.

When they're working properly, deep muscles of the spine actually prevent the vertebrae from collapsing and crushing each other along with the cushioning disks between them. When you unwittingly turn off the main disk-protecting muscles, you're left with a much more vulnerable spine and an increased chance for serious injury, with disk failure being one. The larger muscle groups at the surface of the torso are designed for power and to generate movement. They are different from the spinal stabilizers in that they need to be able to rest some of the time. So, when we rest they rest, and when we move they move. The spinal stabilizers are better at staying active for long periods of time because their job is to work when we are relatively still. Sitting still, standing still; the deep stabilizers are working hard behind the scenes *preventing* and *controlling* our motion instead of making movement happen.

When reflex inhibition has turned off our small, deep spine stabilizers (after a perceived strain), the result is a crushing vice-like effect by the large muscle movers, clumsily trying to help out. This back-up plan can work for a short time to keep us somewhat functional, but it's one of the reasons it can feel so exhausting and uncomfortable to have a back sprain. It becomes an athletic event to simply go about your daily activities. The muscles designed for bursts of energy followed by periods of rest end up instead working overtime with no rest at all until we lie down.

When you find yourself having everyday pain, you have to assume that reflex inhibition is at play, and it becomes essential that you not demand that your spine deal with any potentially unnecessary destabilizing activities. The stabilizers are on hiatus and you are at greater risk of injury while they're "away." Aside from bending forward, the effort involved in lifting your head and torso up off the floor or out of bed can be one of the most stressful things your back has to deal with if you're in pain. Since the protective deep spinal muscles have checked out and your big mover muscles are in control now, any movement you make has a much stronger compressive effect on the joints of the injured areas.

I ask my patients to seriously consider permanently changing the way they move when transitioning from lying to sitting or standing whether there is pain or not. Not only do we never know for sure if our stabilizers are "all systems go" at all times, but there's another dynamic at play with our larger, more superficial, movement muscles that you need to be aware of.

The majority of everyday back or neck pain, at some level, involves a power struggle between the muscle groups that run along the front of the body ("flexors") and the opposing muscles along the back of the body ("extensors").[13] Without dispute, every time these two rival groups go up against each other in a contest, the muscles in the front of the body—the flexors—will win (Figures 5.7 to 5.9).

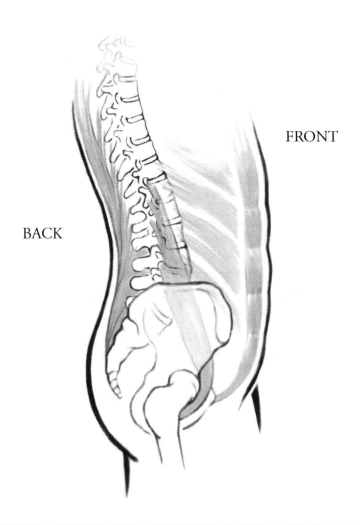

FRONT

BACK

FIGURE 5.7 TORSO FLEXORS VS. EXTENSORS: Flexors are in the front of the torso. The extensors run along the back of the torso.

---

13. Some of you may know that not all extensors are on the back of the body and not all flexors are on the front of the body; however, because the majority are, for the purpose of our discussion of the spine I'll keep it simple.

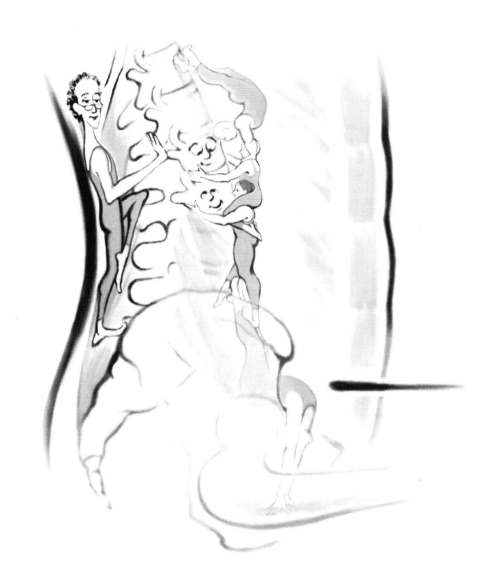

FIGURE 5.8 TORSO FLEXORS AND EXTENSORS BALANCED IN HARMONY: The extensors are often lean and long. The flexors are designed to be short and stout.

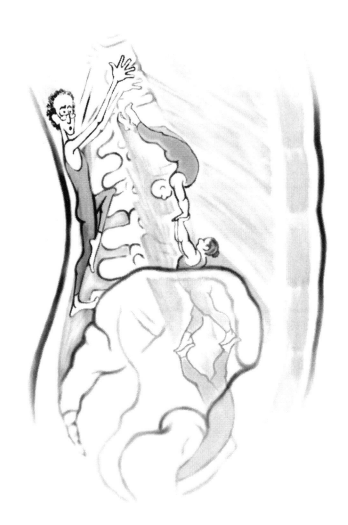

FIGURE 5.9 WHEN THE EXTENSORS (BACK MUSCLES) GET NERVOUS: When reflex inhibition is at play, the extensors on the surface are also more likely to be on edge with even the slightest sensation of pull from the front flexors. This is what can cause over-reactive back tightness as part of our early warning system to let us know that our muscle work load is out of balance.

The flexors along the front of your torso have two very powerful influences working in their favor: gravity and shortness.

You see, it's not strength that wins the fight—it's *force*. A force is a push or pull upon an object resulting from the object's interaction with another object.[14] The bones of the spine are negotiating push and pull between each other every minute of the day. Each vertebra relates to its neighbor vertebrae above and below based on a variety of forces placed on it. When the spine is upright and at relative rest, one of the primary forces on the bones is that of gravity—a compressive force

"When we intentionally stretch the muscle in distress, we are often re-creating exactly one or all of the stressors that this poor muscle thinks it's helping us with in the first place."

exerting influence from the top down. This compressive pressure of gravity can either be magnified or minimized by the action of our muscles. Shortened muscles, regardless of their actual strength, can exert significant forces on the opposing structure that they connect to, simply because they happen to be short and compact (Figure 5.10).

The closer that two objects are to each other, the easier it is to move them even closer. It takes a lot more effort and energy to move two objects together if they are far apart. Just imagine trying to push two pieces of furniture together. For this same reason, any activity against gravity where you find yourself rounding forward/curling or actively contracting muscles in the front of the body, you can be sure that you are adding to the flexors' already excellent ability to pull the body forward, thereby making your back muscles work that much harder to keep you from falling forward and onto your face (Figure 5.11).

---

14. Whenever there is an interaction between two objects, there is a force upon each of the objects. When the interaction ceases, the two objects no longer experience the force. Forces only exist as a result of interaction.

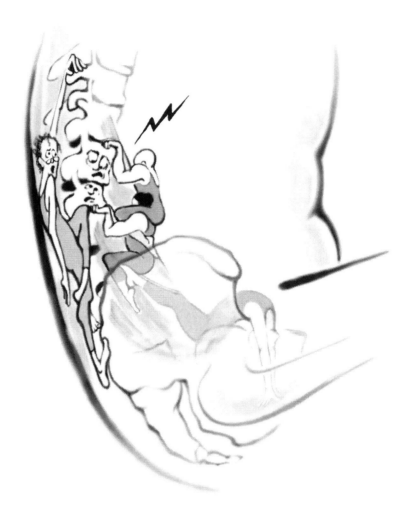

FIGURE 5.10 WHEN THE FLEXORS WIN: This is the actual structural impact of any movement or position that brings your knees closer to your chest, including sitting, curling up on your side to sleep, climbing stairs, sit ups or bending over. When everything is in harmony, we can accommodate for these temporary situations. But if we are injured or simply experiencing reflex inhibition triggered by prolonged poor posture from one-sided tasks, then these everyday situations can cause real problems.

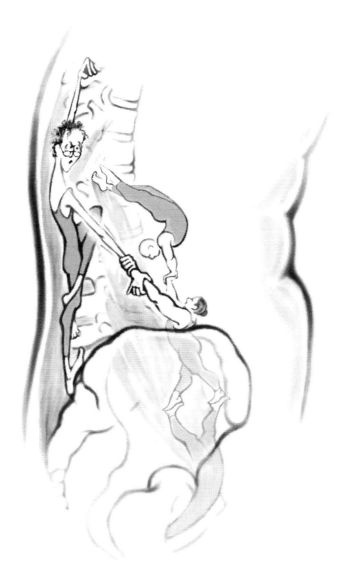

FIGURE 5.11 IMPACT ON YOUR FLEXORS AND EXTENSORS WHEN SLOUCHING: The extensors, our back muscles, are largely preoccupied with keeping us from falling forward in response to the very robust pull by the front flexors—bolstered by hardwired protective reflexes that easily trump the mission of our hard-working back muscles.

Another interesting aspect that feeds into this dominance by the flexor muscles along the front of the torso is a feature that is neurologically hardwired in all of us.

There is a very important protective mechanism called the flexor reflex.[xxiii] The flexor reflex keeps us alive in an emergency by activating some or all of our flexor muscle groups without us first having to think it over. A reflex is by definition an action that results from signals that bypass cognitive areas in the brain—the places where we formulate conscious thought and decision making. We don't have time to weigh options and think things through in cases where reflexes are needed. It's an unconscious process for survival. For example, if your hand accidentally touches a hot stovetop, generally you'll pull your hand back before considering the details of what, why, when and how.

It's the clever flexor reflex that makes this sort of arm recoil possible.[xxiv] Similarly, if you step on a sharp tack with your bare foot, the leg and hip will do the same sort of protective move before you have time to assess what's happening (Figure 5.12A and 5.12B).

To help you picture the scope of our flexor reflex, suppose all of your flexor muscles were maximally activated at the same time; you would find yourself in a fetal position (Figure 5.13). The ultimate protective stance looks like this: head tucked with legs and arms pulled tight into the chest. Think of the "brace for impact" position that airlines advocate for in case of crash landings—same shape. The fetal position will optimally protect your vital organs from injury or attack. A very sensible protective mechanism indeed!

An interesting aside that will be revisited when we look again at the role of emotional stress on pain is the fact that the primitive brain is constantly on the lookout for hazards that might require activation of this flexor reflex. Any time the nervous system is in a heightened state of excitement due to stress, some small aspect of our fight or flight response is triggered. Both fighting and fleeing in the face of danger would require bursts of power to the flexor muscles in particular. Getting to the root of a chronic slouching problem *may* have to start with the question, "Do I feel safe?"

What is really happening to your spine—Scenario 1:

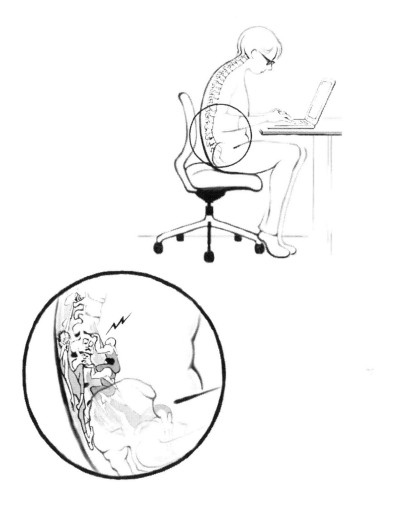

FIGURE 5.12A PROLONGED SITTING FROM THE POINT OF VIEW OF YOUR SPINE: Prolonged sitting in a rounded or straight spine position causes stress that can trigger "reflex inhibition," which turns off the deep spinal stabilizers. When the deep spinal stabilizers are asleep, the large flexors and extensors engage. They try to help but both groups are big and clumsy. The flexors always win the struggle for dominance. When the flexors overpower the extensors in the absence of spinal stabilization by the multifidi, you end up with extremely cranky spinal joints and disks.

What is really happening to your spine—Scenario 2:

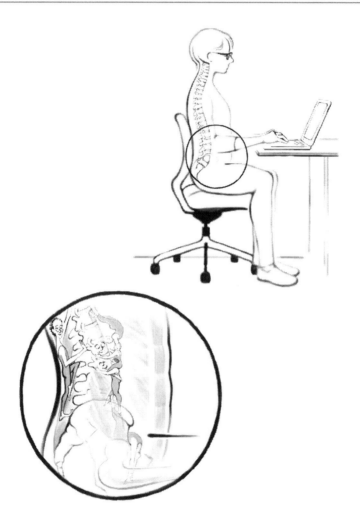

FIGURE 5.12B SITTING—BEST CASE SCENARIO FROM THE POINT OF VIEW OF YOUR SPINE: To keep everyone (the flexors, the extensors and the spinal stabilizers with joints and disks) happy, set your spine up for success and let it sit in the curvy neutral shape it was designed to be in. A gentle supported sway in the lower back is what your spine needs for the least amount of work load in a situation that is less than ideal but that we all have to do every day.

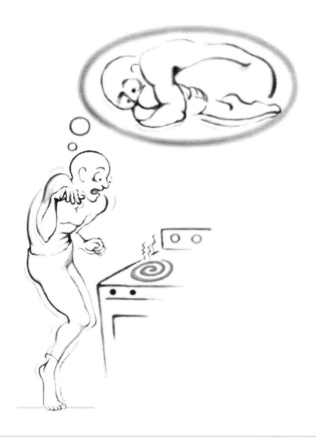

FIGURE 5.13 THE FLEXOR REFLEX SURVIVAL MECHANISM: The "flexor reflex" is one of many survival mechanisms designed to protect us from harm. It's named for the group of muscles that, when maximally activated, create the appearance of what is known as the fetal position.

It follows then that the flexor reflex lines of communication can be buzzing at a low level, on stand-by, to keep the appropriate muscles primed and braced while the brain tries to ascertain the nature of the risk. In the case of protracted (prolonged) stress and anxiety, this means our flexors can develop and hold tension for inordinate amounts of time as they lie in wait for what *might* be just around the corner.

Prolonged tension that is associated with the generalized stress of living can cause chronic shortening and *adhesion* in all of those muscles,[xxv] whose role it is to pull us into a fetal position when necessary.

An adhesion is an area of sticky tissue in and around a muscle with the resultant effect imitating that of shrink wrap (recall Figure 2.8). The purpose of an adhesion is to provide "tensile" strength in an area where there isn't enough muscle tolerance for the chronic stretch it's experiencing. "Tensile" strength refers to the resistance necessary to withstand a pulling-apart kind of pressure. It's a form of structural reinforcement. In order to serve this specific purpose of protecting against a lengthening stress caused by prolonged stretch, the nature of an adhesion has to be rigid, which then renders the tissue in question less flexible and less yielding. Less flexible and less yielding translate into more effective resistance against the force imposed by chronic pulling.

This pulling and struggling to hold on that is experienced by the lengthening muscle groups—commonly along the back of the body—are often generated by, and in response to, the opposite group of muscles that tend to be the short flexor, fetal position muscles—generally along the front of the body. There's really no contest when the flexors of the body grab hold—they are designed to succeed, and this dynamic sets us up for an impossible fight as we struggle to stay upright against gravity. What we're fighting is more than gravity; it's age-old programming in our reptilian brain about survival.

Consider These Two Facts Now:

1. The muscles in the front of our body—by their natural short-ness, together with the pull of gravity itself—easily exert a significant forward rounding force on our skeleton.
2. The protective flexor reflex is by design always at the ready, on a moment's notice, to clamp down and bring us into a fetal position.

With all of these dynamics at play between the front and the back of the body, doesn't it seem like the deck is stacked heavily against our poor back muscles? They are left with the work of holding us upright by constantly pulling the spine back to neutral—all in an effort to keep us from falling forward unopposed. The majority of everyday back pain is the result of one or more groups of back muscles trying to tell us that they have reached their limit for dealing with the imbalance resulting from this force pulling them forward. This means that the last thing these back muscles need is for us to put any more demand on them by choosing activities and positions that put the torso in a rounded position either actively or passively, intentionally or unintentionally.

Stop the Lengthening!

In your quest to stop the pain, hopefully it's becoming clear why it's important to avoid any further shortening of the already dominant short and tight muscles (Figure 5.14). However, it's equally—if not more—essential to prevent any lengthening of the widely under-recognized, already over-lengthened muscle groups, which are struggling against the domineering short muscles causing us to round and curl forward.

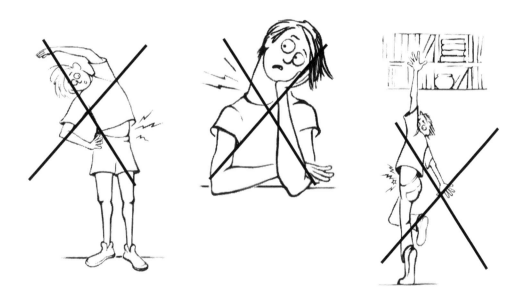

FIGURE 5.14 STOP STRETCHING YOUR PAIN "AWAY"—ELIMINATE THE LENGTHENING STRESS: Stop stretching out the pain to avoid the second of three mechanical stressors on your spine.

> "We nourish our joints by pushing fluids and gases back and forth through movement."

All the muscles that are stressed from being elongated are usually the source of our discomfort. What this means for you if you're in pain is that you need to immediately stop stretching the area that hurts!

(pause) "…What?! But, what if I feel relief when I stretch?"

Unfortunately, all you are doing when you stretch painful and stiff muscles is perpetuating the pain–inflammation cycle. The reason a muscle spasms begin to hurt is because at some point the muscle was pulled past its "acceptable" length (according to your individual neuromechanical blueprint) and now it's overcompensating and rebounding in an attempt to correct the situation. So, stretching what has, more likely than not, been already *overstretched* is just like repeatedly picking away at a scab—not giving it a chance to heal. Stretching *seems* like a good idea because it feels initially helpful, because very often this kind of pain is accompanied by the sensation of stiffness. That spasm is in fact an extreme shortening reaction accompanied by legitimate stiffness. So you ask yourself, "What could be more reasonable than to stretch an area that feels stiff?"

The question should be: What was it that made this muscle or group of muscles feel so threatened that it needed to hunker down so severely? I can guarantee you that it was a lengthening stressor. In the absence of other disease, the muscle tightening of everyday pain is usually a rebound reaction to something that registered in your brain as an inappropriate stretch. It may or may not seem obvious to us, but it's what the brain and nervous system perceive that matters. Going back to what we saw in Chapters 1 and 2 about tissues under stress, remember that lengthening forces are the second of three basic mechanical stressors—an inflammation trigger. Stretching puts a muscle under stress.[xxvi] End of story. So do *not* give in to that urge to stretch. Leave it alone!

If you do stretch that muscle in spasm, you are basically telling it that the tightening over-reaction is indeed justified. Remember, the reason muscles grab and get tight is because they are doing their best to protect you from disaster. Usually that "disaster" is a lengthening, twisting or compressing stress occurring somewhere in the spine and detected by our muscular early warning system.[15] Unfortunately, when we intentionally stretch the muscle in distress, we are often re-creating exactly one or all of the stressors that this poor muscle thinks it's helping us with in the first place.

Not too long after you're done with that stretch, your muscle will go right back to being in spasm because it just received confirmation from you that something is unstable and it had better hold on tight in case that happens again! Stretching the things that hurt actually only feeds the fire and gives the tissues another reason to be and stay inflamed, which is what we experience as painful tension.[16]

Another potential problem in severe cases is that the tight muscle may in fact be acting as a splint in an attempt to keep us from doing more serious damage. If that's the case, then stretching could result in serious consequences because the temporary loosening of that muscular splint might take away the main safety mechanism that is keeping at bay the full impact of a sprain or—worst case scenario—a fracture we didn't know was there. Of course, this would be an extreme instance, and if you have a fracture—even if you didn't yet know it—you wouldn't be calmly reading this book.

Naturally you might be wondering, "Why does the stretch feel so good then?"

As it turns out, there's a very good reason. Because of how we are wired, it is easier to overwhelm the brain with information about the sensation of *stretch* rather than *pain*. Nerves that carry pain sensation are about five times smaller in diameter than the ones that carry stretch sensation.[xxvii] It's like the difference between a five-lane super highway and a dirt country road. The highway will always move much more traffic and much more quickly. So, because stretch sensation moves along the super highway, it dominates. Pain can only move as fast as that one-lane little dirt road.

---

15. The early warning system is in place to preserve vital functioning of our spinal cord and brain, which seems like a good thing to have, but it doesn't always seem to make sense to us because it can deliver *very* early warnings long before those vital structures are truly at risk.

16. None of this applies for the large-scale calf and foot cramping that can happen in the middle of the night. This sort of charley horse spasm needs to be stretched! Cramping is completely different from the tightness at play with everyday pain.

By the time pain makes it up to the brain, if there's a stretch happening at the same time, the brain is already full of stretch sensation and that's all we feel. Because of this phenomenon, when we create a stretch sensation in a muscle that hurts, we temporarily turn off the pain.

This is just one of many examples in life of how what feels good is definitely not always good for you. Stretching a muscle that hurts is just another feel-good, quick fix not unlike the mechanism behind having a cocktail to relax or a cup of coffee to wake up. They all work to a degree but can have unintended consequences and aren't getting to the root of the problem. They—just like stretching—can also be habit-forming long after the behavior stops working.

There are more effective long-term options that will be explored in *Volume Two: Fix the Fire Damage* and *Volume Three: Plan For Fire Prevention* respectively.

Stop the Shearing!

The third source of mechanical stress that was introduced in Chapter 1 is *shearing*. Shearing forces result from combining compression and tension. Compression is what happens when two structures are *squished* together. Tension is the pressure experienced when a structure is *pulled* to its limits. The most common way in which our body experiences compression and tension at the same time is by twisting. Not just twisting alone but twisting while sitting or standing—where gravity and the weight of our own body provides the compression. Additionally, twisting while sitting *and bending* adds a lengthening stretch to the twisted joints, and this combination can push the physiological limits of spinal joints in a hurry if we're not careful. Shearing is one of the most common ways in which spinal disks become stressed. They are actually really well engineered to withstand a great deal of compression. But once you add some twisting to that compression, you start to really push your luck.

This means that when we are trying to make pain stop, not only should we first lie down to eliminate compression and, second, avoid purposefully stretching, but, also consider twisting to be off limits for a little while. Twisting is a form of stretching, so you may already have guessed this, but there are also many normal daily movements that require twisting. Until you're in pain it's easy to miss this (Figure 5.15). One example of a twist in everyday life is checking your blind-spot in the car while driving. Turning over in bed provides a shearing stress as well. Even the rolling I recommend (as part of the stop, drop and roll technique) to safely get yourself up from lying down can impose *some* twisting/shearing stress if you're not careful.

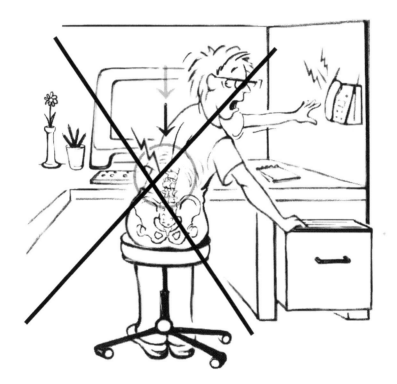

FIGURE 5.15 STOP TWISTING AND REACHING—ELIMINATE THE SHEARING STRESS: Turning and reaching need to stop completely to avoid causing shearing—the third of three mechanical stressors that contribute to the pain and inflammation of everyday pain.

There's a bad habit we all learn as kids in the classroom from being forced to sit in terrible generic chairs for hours on end while stooped over desks that are at the wrong height for many of us. The most natural reaction to this absurd situation is to seek relief by moving or stretching, and when getting up out of the chair doesn't seem like an option, it doesn't take long to find that grabbing on to the back of the chair with both hands and pulling our spines into a twisting stretch gives us relief. It feels relaxing compared with the strain of sitting, but this maneuver is one of the riskier things you can do to your spine, given what we know about how stressful the combination of compression and lengthening (shearing) can be. As with all of our bad habits, the young body is much more tolerant of this kind of stress, but it's another one of many less-than-ideal stressors that we cannot get away with so easily as tissues become less elastic, sometimes with (chemical changes of) age and sometimes because of injuries and their cumulative effect on us over time.

Now, what about twisting yoga poses? Good question. Yoga should be good for you, right? Yes and no. Again, it's a question of balance and individual tolerance for stress, whether that be mechanical, chemical or emotional. If we're talking strictly about the mechanics of the yoga spinal twist, there is definitely some inherent risk due to the shearing stress potential. *If* the back is not in a vulnerable or injured state and *if* the twist is performed with purely muscular effort by the spinal and trunk muscles, only then is it not quite as risky. But if there's encouragement to use your arms by pressing them against your legs or the floor for an added push into a deeper twist, then you're being asked to flirt with disaster.

By making the act of twisting a primarily muscular effort by the spine (without the help of your arms or legs), then we're helping to strengthen the muscles that protect and stabilize the spine and this can be very safe and rehabilitative. The other important piece that allows us to avoid risk with a yoga spinal twist is attention to maintaining a *neutral spine*.

Remember from Figure 2.10 (Chapter 2) that a neutral spine isn't actually straight but instead strategically curved in very specific ways. This includes the presence of a gentle *sway* in the lower back. To maintain that sway during a spinal twist you will need to pay attention to relaxing your belly a bit while allowing the buttocks to protrude toward the back side. Take a look at a toddler's standing spinal shape and you'll see the perfect lower back shape.

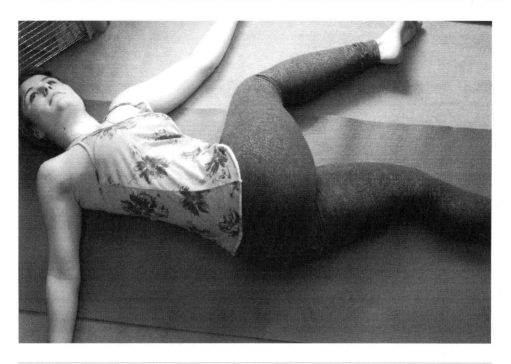

PHOTO 5.4A SPINAL TWIST WITH MORE ROUNDING and less neutral spine can cause subtle mechanical stress that could be avoided by maintaining a neutral spine

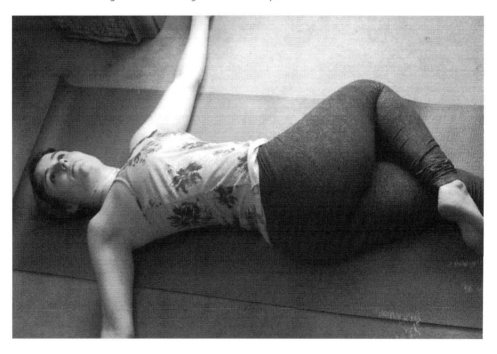

PHOTO 5.4B SPINAL TWIST WITH NEUTRAL SPINE: Notice the gentle lower back sway intact.

If you manage to keep a neutral spine in the lower back (where most of the twisting should be happening) and use only your muscular effort, then the spinal twist you achieve may feel like barely five degrees of rotation, but you'll be coming by it honestly. If that is all your muscles can do for you in that moment, then that is all the rotation you should get. This might be a good time to implement the practice of embracing the idea that less is more. It really can be. So, above all, don't force it!

Something that happens for many people when they force their back to twist is that they experience some cracking and popping in the spine. One of the most common questions I hear from patients about treatment is, "What *is* that? What's making that noise?" People especially want to know this if I'm the one causing this noise in their spine with treatment. The cracking of the spine is a topic that is cloaked in confusion and urban myths. To many people it sounds and feels like something is breaking or as though bones are rubbing together. Neither of those things is happening. Because it usually gets a giggle, I like to explain to my very young patients: it's not all that dissimilar to what happens when we noisily pass gas. Yes, you read that right.

The cracking noise of a joint is the result of an exchange of gases between what is a pressurized system inside of our joint capsules and the environment outside of and next to the joint—the body tissues.[xxviii] Gases are constantly being exchanged between joints and body tissues with our everyday movements. We nourish our joints by pushing fluids and gases back and forth through movement.

Every joint has a bubble around it—the joint capsule. Inside of this capsule is a pressurized system. It's a somewhat separate compartment from the rest of the body tissues because it needs to maintain an environment unique to the needs of the joint. To ensure smooth movement we need lubrication around the movable joints, and it just so happens that there is a special fluid, "synovial fluid," for that purpose. It's one of the main things we keep inside of that pressurized joint bubble. Pressurization, along with these joint fluids, provides us with lubrication and cushioning in motion. The capsule that surrounds the joint is permeable to some degree, but it's firm and thereby provides the barrier necessary to maintain these special needs of the joint.

When full movement is reintroduced into a joint that has not moved through its full potential range for a little while,[17] the capsule experiences outside pressure, is forced to deform a little to accommodate this pressure and the resulting differential pushes its way across the capsule more quickly than usual, from inside to out and outside to in. Sometimes there's a cracking/popping noise because of this and sometimes there isn't. The noise or lack of noise depends on the body chemistry and level of systemic inflammation, which is why not everyone's joints do pop and crack.

And, "how," you ask yourself, "is this similar to passing gas?!"

- When there's gas buildup in your gut, sometimes you feel the pressure and sometimes you don't. When your joints are restricted/jammed, sometimes you feel the pressure and sometimes you don't.
- When the gas builds up enough and becomes trapped there can be pain. When the joints get badly stuck enough there can be pain.
- When the gas in your gut finally moves and escapes, sometimes it makes noise and sometimes it doesn't. When full joint motion is restored or a restriction is freed up, sometimes it makes noise and sometimes it doesn't.
- When intestinal gas is released it can bring incredible relief. When stuck joints are released it also can bring incredible relief.

So, you see, despite how it sounds, nothing is actually breaking apart or rubbing together when that crack happens. Pressure, gases and molecules are shifting. Among the many other powerful effects of a true joint crack (or "cavitation," as it's technically called), endorphins and other painkilling chemicals are released due to the stimulation of the tissues immediately surrounding the joint. This is one of the reasons it can feel so good to receive a spinal adjustment *and* it's why many people develop a craving for the quick fix of that relieving sensation. Unfortunately, there can definitely be too much of this good thing—especially when it becomes a craving

---

17. Recall from Chapter 1 the discussion about excess motion in the joints and how that can cause a protective decrease in motion or a locking up of *neighboring* joints and muscles.

that is followed by repeated self-administered cracks in an attempt to get that quick fix feeling. If this sounds like you, then you need to understand that this is *not at all* a safe thing to do to yourself.

Sometimes cracking and popping can just happen without intention as we go about our daily business and that is usually not something to worry about. It does, however, indicate that your spine is handling an uneven workload and probably needs some form of manual therapy to restore full and balanced motion. From my point of view, it's one of those early warning system hints the body gives us to go get a professional spinal adjustment/alignment/correction. But if you are someone who forcefully makes your own back or neck crack several times a day and to the point where it has become a habit, so much so that you don't even think about or notice it anymore, then you should at least be aware of how very bad this can be for you.

First of all, when we try to get a joint to pop on our own body, we have to use long levers to do so. Unfortunately, we can't just reach around and press on one specific spot. Using long levers usually means we are creating length between two far away points in order to get that pop to happen. (Remember what was said in Chapter 2 about lengthening being one of the three main mechanical triggers of inflammation.) Think about that twisting around in the chair example. Not only does lengthening provide an inflammatory trigger—a primary mechanical stressor—but by doing it this way we usually are only accessing and affecting the joint capsule that will pop with the least amount of effort. It's the first area to yield.

Joint cracking will always give us short-lived relief because of the chemical reaction created. Endorphins (natural pain-killers) are released from the stimulation at and around the capsule, but the joint that pops with this non-specific stretching maneuver is one that is already hypermobile anyway. It's the weakest link. That's why it's popping so easily. And, if it's being popped repeatedly by you throughout the day, then it's only becoming weaker and more hypermobile, which will signal to all of the surrounding joints and muscles to "hold on!" and "tighten up!" in order to compensate for this now excessive motion. The only thing you're doing when you fall into this self-cracking trap is perpetuating the problem.

The whole reason you're craving that crack or stretch in the first place is because your muscles tightened up. Your body is smart and usually muscles tighten because something is moving *too much* or in the wrong direction. If you continue moving things around too much or in that same wrong direction, you're letting your muscles know that they had better stay tight.

This cycle we can get stuck in with the joint cracking is similar to the itch-scratch cycle. The more you scratch an itch, the itchier it gets. You have to find a way to stop scratching before you break the skin.

When a chiropractor scans for which areas to adjust—where to administer the popping release (associated with some of the traditional techniques)—it's only the joints that are the *most* jammed up that we're looking for. The point is to restore motion at the *real* areas of restriction, which allows the areas that have been moving too much to relax.

The delivery of a spinal adjustment the way chiropractors are trained to do it should be very quick and very specific. It's the speed of the adjustment maneuver that avoids imposing any lengthening stress anywhere. It's also done with short levers, which means movement happens only over a very small area of the body at a time—spanning one or two joints. This makes it extremely specific, in a way that we cannot be with ourselves. With such specificity, a skilled chiropractic treatment introduces movement over a nanosecond of time, only where it's needed and nowhere else. When jammed-up joints are properly released, then those hypermobile joints—the ones that are cracking all the time—should not feel compelled to do so much of the work anymore. The work load becomes more evenly distributed and sensations of tightness will ease.

Once the self-administered cracking has become a daily habit—a dependency—you run the real risk of destroying the tone of your ligaments, which are some of the main stabilizing elements that connect the bones of your spine to each other. If you imagine stripping away all of your muscles, you would see that each bone connects to the other by these non-elastic strands that we call "ligaments." They are made of material that does not have a lot of give and that is because they are there to stabilize the joint—to protect it from too much movement. Repeated forceful cracking will cause these ligaments to stretch out and become loose and unsupportive.

Once we've weakened the ligaments—our most stabilizing structures next to bone—then the muscles of the spine have to work so much harder than they are designed to, on a day-to-day basis, simply to accomplish being upright against gravity. People who constantly, purposefully and forcefully crack their own spinal joints are damaging their support structure and setting themselves up for serious injury down the road.

All of these complications from what seems like a fun and stress-relieving thing to do are just not worth it in the long run. Not to mention that any kind of repeated stimulation to anywhere in the body will cause friction, which can only result in inflammation—just like a blister that forms from the rubbing of a badly fitting shoe. The inflammation may not be felt as pain right away but it will provide the initial spark to what may turn into a situation like a pile of simmering coals that ignites decades later, once we've hit our limit for stress in that area.

Move Like a Robot!

If you are doing things right, you'll notice that the result of stopping or controlling all the different possible mechanical stressors makes you feel incredibly robotic and unnatural:

- You will be holding your head directly over your center at all times.
- You will not be reaching with your arms at any distance away from your body center.
- You'll be using your legs to move up and down so your torso doesn't have to round or pitch forward at all.

That's right, it will feel awkward and silly, but it won't look nearly as odd as it feels, and it's well worth the effort because this is the way to keep any shortening (compressive), lengthening or twisting stresses from affecting your fresh and tender strain or sprain. Giving in to this move-like-a-robot technique will allow your area of pain to recover as quickly as it can without the continual irritation of all the familiar but stressful habits of moving through the day in the routine way. These changes to how you move may seem dramatic if it's new for you, but it's *completely* reasonable to go to the extreme with this sort of early intervention. You're simply being sensible. If you do it now and do it well, it won't be forever.

Just because this is currently the most pain-free way to move in the face of pain does *not* mean that you are forever destined to move like a robot. However, if you choose not to move radically differently and carefully during a time of pain, you are essentially repeatedly picking at a scab, thereby not allowing the repair process to happen properly. Every time you move into the pain of an injury or allow it to happen by letting your guard down, you are getting in the way of the healing process and your recovery will be slower than necessary.

CHAPTER 6

Put Out the Kindling:
Address the Chemical Triggers

THESE CHEMICAL TRIGGERS ARE A LITTLE sneakier than the mechanical category of everyday pain triggers—less obvious, just like glowing embers disguised as white coals: They don't necessarily *look* all that hot or dangerous, but they will easily ignite any nearby kindling in a heartbeat.

If your pain is not completely new, then it's very likely that the initial steps of stopping, dropping and rolling (as was laid out at the beginning of this chapter), are not going to have a very dramatic effect on your situation. These are still steps you should take, because they will help to begin recalibrating the body's sense of where it should physically be occupying space in order to be more comfortable, restoring a sense of "neutral."

Although the relief from the stop, drop and roll technique is temporary, it's an important set of actions needed not only to restore mechanical peace, but also to re-educate your neuroendocrine system (part of what controls body chemistry) about how to *not* be in pain. Any reminder you can give your body of what it was like before there was pain, the better the chances are that you'll be able to get back to that pain-free place sooner.

Unfortunately, the fact is that, after pain has become a familiar part of your everyday life, there are more complex things at play than just the mechanical irritants. When familiar old pain is triggered or flares up, it's usually tightly intertwined with a chemical cascade of inflammatory troublemakers inside of the cells and tissues.[xxix] The best way to address this old sort of familiar pain will be by focusing on breaking the *chemical* pain cycle. When the chemistry of pain and inflammation is under control, it allows for the efforts at structural change to take better effect. Those structural changes are often best achieved with the help of things like physical therapy, strengthening or better attention to neutral posture. If those things are being diligently deployed and the results are less than shining, then it might be time to think about how to deal with the chemical triggers that are often at play behind the scenes and hampering the progress (Figure 6.1).

Ice or Heat?

For both old and new pain, when it spikes or first appears, the initial step should always be to apply ice. I often hear confusion about when and whether to apply ice or heat.

Most simply put:

- Ice is for cooling inflammation
- Heat is for loosening the grip of tight muscles

"Any reminder you can give your body of what it was like before there was pain, the better the chances are that you'll be able to get back to that pain-free place sooner."

Control the Inflammation Traffic Jam!

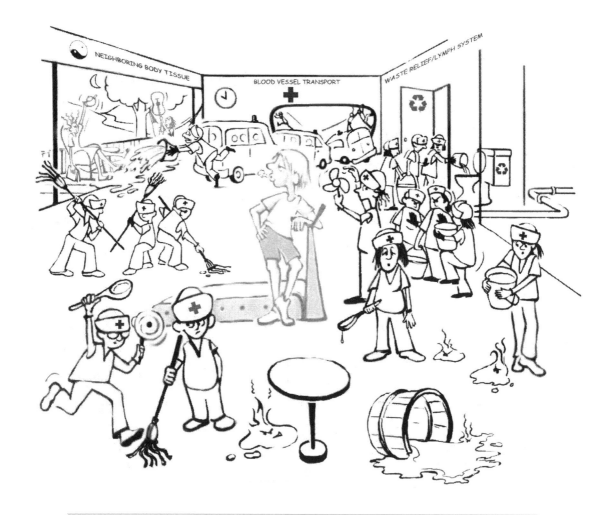

FIGURE 6.1 STOP THE BUILDUP OF WASTE—ELIMINATE THE CHEMICAL IRRITATION CAUSING PAIN: Now that you got off the treadmill and stopped the mechanical stress, the back-up of inflammatory mediators—clean-up crew and tissue waste products—are causing pain and irritation.

Heat *feels* good but can actually slow down tissue repair by keeping the area inflamed. (Again, sadly, what feels good isn't always good for us.) Heat is more often a useful tool in areas that are chronically shortened like all of those flexor muscles along the front of the body that we talked about earlier (in our discussion about the struggle to stay upright against gravity). Heat can help these hard-working, short and tight tissues loosen and lengthen a bit as they relax from the increased blood flow in response to the warming process. Consider placing a hot water bottle on the belly when you have lower back pain or heat over your chest when you have neck or upper back pain. Placing heat on the opposing and often short muscle groups (the regions on the other side of the body from where the pain is) will make the simultaneous application of ice to the back or neck seem much more tolerable and less psychologically unappealing while creating a very complementary effect.

You can safely assume (based on what you've learned in Chapter 1) that when pain first appears or flares up, inflammation is a major factor, which is why applying ice to the area is always a good first step. Be aware that even if your pain is accompanied by the sensation of stiffness, if it's new pain or a new recurrence of old pain, ice may still be a better idea than heat. While heat often feels good and is comforting, it can make inflammation worse.[18] The way that ice works is by squeezing the blood vessels in the area of the injury just like squeezing a hose to narrow the flow of water. This can control the sometimes unruly influx of inflammation helpers—those chemical mediators. After the ice is removed, the blood vessels relax and new flow and drainage is allowed to occur again.

Overall, the benefit of ice application lies equally in the *removal* of the ice pack. So, try not to fall asleep on your ice pack; you'll be negating the effects if it stays cold for too long. It's been proven that intermittent ice applications of 10 minutes each are more effective than one application lasting 20 minutes.[xxx] Repeated applications like this will create a pumping action in the vessels around the area of pain to get helper molecules (aid vehicles and clean-up crew) *in* to the area in need, while waste (broken down tissue and tired, used-up clean-up crew) will be more efficiently moved *out* of the way (Figure 6.2).

---

18. This is in contrast/conflict with the school of thought among Eastern medicine practitioners on heat vs. ice.

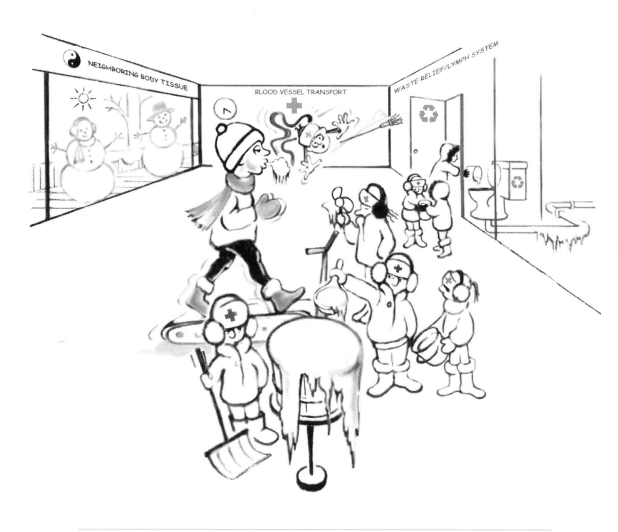

FIGURE 6.2 USE ICE: Applying ice to the area in pain helps by squeezing out the pain-causing chemicals of inflammation.

For various reasons some people's pain can feel worse with ice, and in that case, alternating ice and heat applications can be a good alternative option with a fresh injury, more gently accomplishing the same effect as ice only.[xxxi]

Ice is a great first defense against inflammation pain but it has its limits. It mainly acts locally—just on the area around the injury or wherever you apply it. Very often the long term success of easing inflammation at the site of an injury depends upon the condition of neighboring tissues and in fact requires the help of those healthy unaffected tissues and systems of the body. Total body inflammatory load can significantly impact inflammation coping at the site of pain. Because of this, we want to be sure to address all the different ways in which the body eliminates waste so that the injured area has the best chance of the most efficient recovery possible.

Remember from Chapter 1 that whenever there is pain, there is inflammation. Wherever there is inflammation, there is an increase in waste production. Not only is the extra waste a large part of what causes pain, but the well-meaning cleanup crew that gets automatically recruited to help with the mess is *also* pain producing if they're allowed to linger. Just think of an uncomfortably crowded room of people— even if everyone is there to help, after a certain point it can become too much for everyone. So, if you're looking for relief of *chemically* mediated pain, what you have to do is to escort *all* of these irritants out of the area as efficiently as possible.

There are three main ways by which we can encourage waste elimination from the injured body part:

1. Manually through movement
2. Flushing the area with fluids
3. Controlling inflammation (minimizing or eliminating current levels as well as new sources)

Move It!

Manual movement of pain-causing elements around an injury can be by way of bodywork like massage, chiropractic,[xxxii] or acupuncture.[19,xxxiii] Manual stimulation can also come from simply, carefully and safely introducing movement into the areas around the injury, keeping in mind the need to maintain neutral, stress-free positioning whenever possible. This is why bed rest has long been revealed to actually not be good for back pain. The movement, when done safely, helps to transport the inflammation out and get you back on track sooner.

---

19. Acupuncture acts on many complex levels other than manual stimulation, but it has been shown to have an alleviating effect on inflammation.

Flush It!

Flushing the area under stress to relieve it of chemical irritants can happen in a number of ways (Figure 6.3A). Drinking more water is an easy and effective way to push things through the tissues very basically by adding hydraulic pressure and literally rinsing everything out. Water passes through the body to the kidneys on its way back out via the bladder (Figure 6.3E). The way the fluids get to the kidneys in the first place is by a network of vessels called the "lymphatic system." Lymphatic vessels are like the body's sewage system. They are a network of vessels that move fluid (lymph), carrying garbage out of all the corners of the body (Figure 6.3B). Waste destinations are through the kidneys, out the colon and the pores in our skin (Figure 6.3C). So, we escort trash out with finality by peeing, pooping and sweating—all three of which you can do more easily when you're well hydrated!

Another way to optimize this flushing effect and really to take advantage of your effort at increased water intake is to ingest enzymes and herbs along with the water. There are certain herbs that have been shown to help break down and neutralize the pain-causing molecules of waste and of repair.[xxxiv] These broken down and neutralized molecules would then be escorted out via the elimination portion of the digestive tract—your colon (Figure 6.3D).

Enzymes taken for inflammation should be "full spectrum," meaning they should include all three groups of enzyme types (amylase, proteases, lipases), which together break down carbohydrates, proteins and fats. The molecules of waste and clean-up are made up of all three of these components. In addition to enzymes, three examples of herbs that help to break down inflammation-causing chemicals are turmeric, ginger, and *Boswellia serrata*.[xxxv,xxxvi] All of these are available in supplement form and, even though you can just add turmeric and ginger to your diet, in order to get a therapeutic effect when dealing with painful levels of inflammation, concentrated doses are recommended.[20]

---

20. Always consult with your health care professional before taking any supplement or herb because some of these herbs might not agree well with some people or may be contraindicated in certain conditions or when taken with other medications.

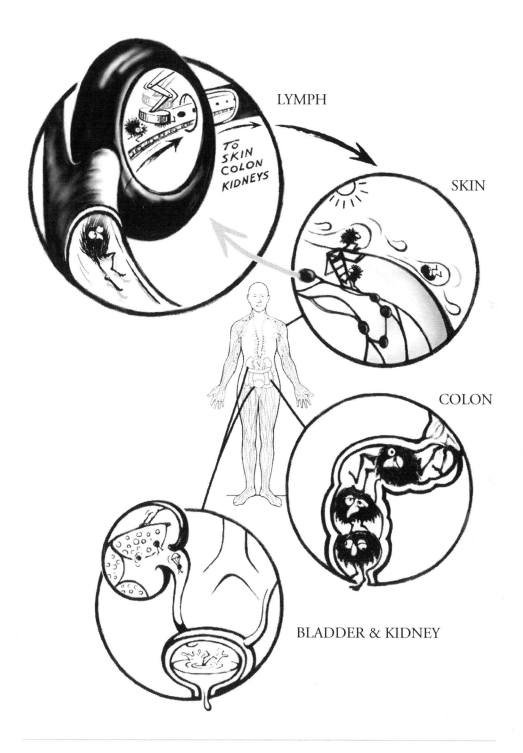

FIGURE 6.3A WASTE-ELIMINATION PATHWAYS: Lymph, skin, colon and kidneys.

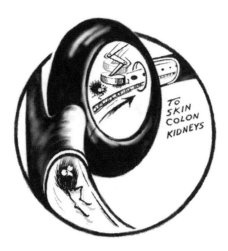

FIGURE 6.3B LYMPHATIC FLUID ("LYMPH"), VESSELS AND LYMPH NODES: Waste gets eliminated via the lymphatic fluid transported through networks of lymphatic vessels not unlike networks of blood vessels. Lymph nodes are like sewage-treatment plants complete with trash compactors strategically placed at intervals along these networks. This is where immune responses are waged against countless microscopic invaders and waste products. Here they are rendered inert and prepared for elimination via sweat, urine and stool.

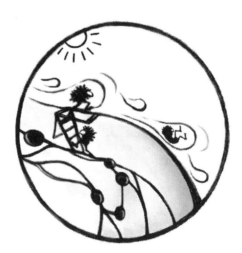

FIGURE 6.3C SKIN AND SWEAT: Waste being eliminated via sweat from the lymph system of vessels out through the skin. This is why dry saunas can be so purifying. Sweating can unburden us from some of our toxin load.

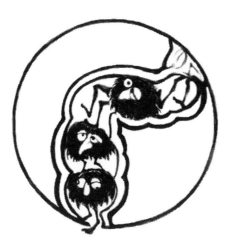

FIGURE 6.3D THE COLON: Waste being eliminated via the colon is often an under-appreciated, daily detoxifying function. Until there's a problem with this system, we don't realize how life-changing that daily routine can be.

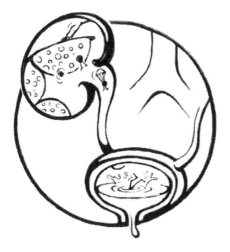

FIGURE 6.3E BLADDER AND KIDNEYS: Waste being eliminated via the bladder and kidneys is very carefully filtered first.

Avoid It!

After all of the hard work of changing your body positioning habits, seeking out the appropriate bodywork treatments and flushing with water and enzymes, you don't want to ruin it all by allowing perfectly avoidable sources of inflammation to continue bogging down your progress. This means you should take care to avoid inflammatory foods, control your stress level as best as you can and get as much sleep as is possible.

Watch Your Inflammatory Food Intake!

There are many resources out now about different approaches to the anti-inflammatory diet. The tricky thing to be aware of here is that not everybody has the same degree of inflammatory response to the same foods. Many so-called food allergies, sensitivities or intolerances are basically inflammatory reactions to proteins within that food. The body regards some proteins as foreign and reacts to them in the same way it would to a virus—it triggers mobilization of the immune response. When the total load on the immune system is under control, we don't usually notice that there's a reaction going on because our body is handling the situation, and allergens (or foreign proteins) are being held in balance with our waste-removal capacity. It's only when systems become overloaded with waste, inflammation and maybe illness that we become unable to cope with the dietary trigger and vice versa.

Some inflammatory reactions to food are because of the substances used to process the food in order to extend shelf life or enhance flavor. Other reactions are from the challenge of handling the pH changes that the food imposes on us. As we spoke of briefly in Chapter 3, some foods cause our body tissues to become more acidic, which creates a welcoming environment for inflammation. A few foods[xxxvii] that are without a doubt inflammation-causing are coffee—even decaffeinated[xxxviii]—alcohol, sugar, simple starches (which just translate to sugar inside the body), animal proteins—red meat most of all—and chemical preservatives such as nitrates, nitrites, sulfates and sulfites. (See The Appendix for further reading.)

Stress & Sleep

It's no mystery that sleep is an essential part of life, but *exactly* why is still a bit of a mystery scientifically speaking. What we do know is how detrimental *lack* of adequate sleep can be, and you don't have to be a scientist to know this. Sleep science is a quickly growing area of study that is revealing how very integral sleep is in regard to everything from memory deficits to heart disease and mental illness. A large part of the underlying side effect of sleep deprivation is inflammation.[xxxix, xl]

Do you recall from Chapter 3 the vicious cycle of stress we can get trapped in because of our brain chemicals? No one *wants* to be stressed, but some of us start to *need* it biochemically in order to simply make it through the day. Stress chemicals like cortisol are actually *anti*-inflammatory, but cortisol is a chemical designed only for short-term use. We should only be relying on cortisol to deal with limited bursts of stress. When we experience, as many of us do, prolonged periods of stress, cortisol outstays its welcome and can lead to lowered immune functioning, high blood sugar, high blood pressure, among many other things—all things that in small bursts for a specific purpose can help the body deal with stress. Obviously, over a longer period of time these chronically elevated cortisol levels outlive their purpose and the conditions resulting from these high sustained levels start causing harm to the body. This mayhem can ultimately result in chronic body-wide inflammation, then depression and subsequently biological addiction to stress as we saw in Diagram 3.2B (Chapter 3).

Knowing that sleep can alleviate stress or help us cope with stress, it's not too much of a leap to imagine that sleep, in turn, can alleviate or prevent inflammation. So, when we are compromised by pain, we know it becomes especially important to review our stress loads at home and at work. But attending to getting as much good quality sleep as possible can be equally instrumental, yet often overlooked, in facilitating repair and recovery of strains and sprains.

> "It's only when systems become overloaded with waste, inflammation and maybe illness that we become unable to cope with the dietary trigger and vice versa."

Now, if you are in the stage of pain that is also disrupting your sleeping position, then you may have to bring the neutral spine, passive-release technique (as part of the stop, drop and roll method from earlier in this chapter) into bed with you until your body can manage some of your favorite sleeping positions without pain again. It's also possible that you'll need to review these options with someone who can advise you on the safety of your positioning for sleep based on your specific situation and discuss whether or not your favorite position is one that you should expect to return to in the future.

What About Over-the-Counter Pain Medication?

We can't complete this chapter on how to stop pain without acknowledgment of widely available over-the-counter medications like ibuprofen, naproxen, aspirin or acetaminophen. We can always choose to turn off the pain with any one of these tools and carry on our merry way. While all pharmaceutical medicine has a time and place, using nonsteroidal anti-inflammatory drugs (NSAIDs) without first exploring the source of pain can be akin to covering up the "check engine" light on the dashboard with a big piece of black tape. It will work to make you feel better until the cause of the check engine light disables other systems and stops you in your tracks again.

Pain medication, either over the counter or as prescribed, can also be a necessary way to break the chemical pain cycle long enough to let the body remember its way back to pre-inflammation status. It can be well worth investigating with the help of a health care expert who knows you and your health history and can help you weigh the question of *when* and *if* medication is the right thing for you. If you are making the choice to use NSAIDs, you should be aware of a few things that may encourage you to be judicious with the questions of how much to take and for how long.

Here are just some of the facts about how NSAIDs can affect you:

- They are known to disrupt the natural enzyme repair process of joints.[xli]
- They are cleared by the body either through the kidneys or the liver, which *can* cause kidney and/or liver stress.[xlii, xliii] This kidney and liver stress can, for some of us, be an issue over time.
- They also are well known for their potentially ulcerative effect on the upper gastrointestinal tract, in some cases causing internal bleeding.[xliv]
- They are being more closely examined for their effect on the cardiovascular system—hypertension being one such effect.[xlv]

In my opinion, if you are aware of the potential drawbacks to any drug or therapeutic intervention, then at least you can make your choices with eyes open and decide for yourself whether or not the benefits outweigh the risks based on your personal needs. If, for a short period of time, you feel the need for pain relief in order to function *and* you make sure to implement as many of the stress-reducing (mechanical, chemical and emotional) tactics as you can, then you shouldn't feel guilty about your choice to use medication. If it is done with moderation and goal setting, then hopefully you won't get stuck depending on it. If you stop the medication and the pain comes right back, then you haven't done what you need to do to fix the stressors. Do more than just cover up your check engine light when it becomes a bother for you to have to look at it. Check the engine. Fix the problem.

What if it's Not Just Everyday Pain?

"Everyday" pain is the kind of pain that is not permanent. It's caused by specific mechanical, chemical and emotional triggers—triggers that you can change and control. This kind of pain will respond and improve once you address one or all three of these triggers.

It should certainly be noted that if you are trying all of the sensible ways to eliminate the triggers in your life but the pain is either not changing or not getting progressively better, then your body is probably in a state of inflammation beyond your control. There may be a different, more complex underlying cause for your inflammation because of another condition you may or may not know about. When there is a disease process like rheumatoid arthritis, diabetes or endometriosis, it becomes much more difficult for you to find any lasting relief from the simple aches of an unrelated strain of the everyday variety with the basic methods presented here in this book. It's not impossible, but doing so will take much more patience and understanding on your part once you get help from your doctor, who is the one who can find out what's really going on.

Remember: If nothing makes your pain feel better, don't wait. Get help. See a doctor right away.

Dampen the Emotional Flame: Attend to the Mental Triggers

Above all, don't panic!

This is easier said than done, but if you follow my suggestions in Section II by taking the steps to stop the mechanical triggers and take control of the chemical triggers, you will prove to yourself that there really is nothing to panic about. If you can decrease the pain *even just by a little bit*, by either lying down or putting ice on it, for example, then that's solid proof that things are not hopeless. It's just going to take some patience and a change in your expectations of your body while it does its best to get better.

By addressing the mechanical and chemical factors of your pain, you take control and show yourself that this is something you can affect and have control over. If you try all these things and there is no change in your pain, then by all means, panic.[21] But, most of the time you'll find that the pain and limitation that you're experiencing is a perfectly reasonable response by your body to a common stressor that it has been trying to manage for years without telling you and now it's just reached its limit. This is especially true of pain that seems to come out of nowhere or that feels to you as though the pain reaction is way out of proportion from what seems to have caused the pain—like brushing your teeth or washing the dishes or just sleeping—of all things!

Remember, stress hormones increase inflammation over the long term (Diagram 3.2B in Chapter 3). So, how you handle the stress around this everyday pain will either lengthen or speed up your recovery.

Aside from the initial panic of the "what the heck is going on?!" reaction to pain, the next most common emotional struggle encountered when dealing with nagging and recurring bouts of everyday pain is that of feeling defective. The "am I broken?" funk hits hard when comparing your current situation with that teenage or preteen carefree self of yours or maybe even your very sensible self of just yesterday. Having the experience and comparison of any times when your body seemed unstoppable can make it so much harder to accept the current situation. It's especially hard to see the current bout of pain without harsh judgment or feelings of defeat.

The "am I broken?" funk quickly leads to deeper angst about our limited time in this body. So, while you're trying your best to avoid panicking, remember that yes, you are growing older and your body is therefore less tolerant of *some* behavior than it used to be, but this is not the beginning of the end. This is only a temporary glitch. You're experiencing a redirect (sometimes, unfortunately, a very painful one), and no matter how well you think you already take care of yourself, there's usually something that can change in response to this incident of unexpected pain that will show you what. Be open to learning new ways to be well in the body you have.

Your everyday pain can be the beginning of a new phase of positive change and,

---

21. Joking aside, if you truly can't find any changes in your pain, then it's important to seek help from a health care professional.

> "A large part of the underlying side effect of sleep deprivation is inflammation."

thanks to the pain, you can no longer ignore the fact that it might simply be time to reconfigure either the physical, chemical or emotional demands on your body. Maybe it's time to look at where you can make changes in your life to support better and more consistent self-care, whether it's scheduling time or budgeting money for daily or weekly moments to breathe, walk or exercise. Maybe it's about figuring out how to kindly say no to people or situations in your life so that you stop giving away that time that you need for your own emotional health and energy. Maybe you've already done these things but recently fell away from some of it and you just need to rededicate to it. In this case, be kind to yourself and realize that it's okay and simply human nature to fall out of our good habits. Let yourself start over again and do what you know works for you, whether it's going to bed early, making better food choices or getting outside more often.

One tricky thing is to watch that self-care doesn't end up feeling like a punishment to you. Taking care of yourself is something you *deserve*.

Something you should keep in mind when fighting the worry that things might be hopeless: As long as we have living tissue to work with, there really is always potential for change! Nothing that is living is static and that is the one thing we are always guaranteed in life—for better or for worse. In the case of finding our way out of everyday pain, I choose for better! I hope you do too.

SUMMARY:
Section II — How Do I Make it Stop?

Control the Traffic Jam to Control the Pain

Pain and Inflammation = Build-Up of Triggers (traffic jam)

Stop all the inflammatory behavior
Drop and lie down! Take a load off
Roll, don't sit straight up after lying down

STOP THE MECHANICAL TRIGGERS:
(GET OFF THE "TREADMILL")

- ✓ Lie down to avoid compression
- ✓ Avoid stretching
- ✓ Avoid twisting

STOP THE CHEMICAL TRIGGERS:
(CLEAR THE "TRAFFIC JAM")

- ✓ Apply ice or heat
- ✓ Get or give yourself gentle manual therapy
- ✓ Flush your body with water/hydrate
- ✓ Clean up with enzymes and herbs
- ✓ Avoid additional chemically stressful food

SUMMARY:

(Continued)

STOP THE EMOTIONAL TRIGGERS:
(CHANNEL THE "PEACEFUL NEIGHBOR" VIBE)

- ✓ Stress control
- ✓ Sleep
- ✓ Don't panic

Section III

How Do I Keep it From Happening Again?

CHAPTER 7

Make Yourself Fire Proof!
(physically, chemically and emotionally)

AFTER THE PAIN FROM THE FIRE of inflammation subsides and you find yourself moving about more easily again, it will be very tempting to simply return to life as usual with a big sigh of relief. After all, you probably have a ton of things to catch up on after being laid up with your unexpected episode of this very disruptive, albeit everyday kind of pain. When being forced to take it easy because of this sort of thing, you can't help but let some responsibilities slide while focusing on getting better. But before you return to autopilot, you should know that this is a *crucial* time. Right now is when the memory of your strain is still fresh, and yet you aren't completely hindered by it anymore. *This* is the time when you need to explore some different ways to move forward, not just mechanically, but chemically and emotionally too. Do it before you lose the valuable feedback that the slight remaining pain can offer you.

A familiar saying comes to mind here, about the definition of insanity being: "to do the same thing over and over while expecting different results." Yet we've all been guilty of that at some stage in our lives, haven't we? It's especially easy to ignore the need for change when it's not entirely clear *what* needs to change in the first place. One thing's for sure, though; we can't continue doing what we've been doing without expecting identical results. It will just be a matter of time before we find ourselves in the exact same situation and possibly even worse. In fact, after the initial injury we become much more vulnerable to *re*-injury if we don't make sure to change something.[xlvi]

Remember, pain often appears the same way a bucket suddenly spills over, even though it may have been filled to the brim for a long time. All it takes is one last tiny drop into that brimming bucket, and so, all we remember is that one last drop which pushed things over the edge. We don't always realize what all those other things were that gradually and slowly filled that bucket to the brim in the first place, but it's these contributing stressors that we have to learn about so we can avoid filling that bucket too full again.

If you're reading through the chapters in sequence, you probably see by now that pain and inflammation are usually the result of a cumulative effect like this, caused by many different types of triggers— mechanical, chemical and emotional in nature— all acting together. So, how *do* we figure out where to begin, in order to keep it from happening again? The first step is to become inflammation—"fire proof"—mechanically, chemically *and* emotionally. Eliminate the risk of igniting hot simmering coals that you don't know are there, by ensuring that you are not providing a welcome environment for those simmering coals in the first place.

For starters, it's very important to discover which stressors are the hottest button triggers for *your* body in particular. What specific situation pushes *you* most easily to the edge and produces pain by playing on these weak spots that are specific to *your* body? Everyone has his or her own unique vulnerabilities for stress in all three areas (mechanical, chemical and emotional), and determining what yours are can take some time. Your individual stressors can also change with age and circumstance, which is why it's always a good idea to take inventory after each episode, while the pain is subsiding.

Check in with what you thought was working and find out why it hasn't. Are your weak spots changing or was the stressor/trigger a little different from anything your body has ever had to deal with? Maybe it was a familiar and repetitive trigger— it just happened one time too many. The first few times you try this sort of troubleshooting, you may do better with some outside help from your care provider of choice. Someone who has worked with your body and who knows your typical points of restriction or imbalance can help you gain better perspective with the benefit of his or her outside vantage point.

The path toward becoming fire-proof involves some
fine tuning: Do you remember Ed?

ED is my patient who hurt himself reaching for the toothpaste. So long as he is able to take extra care to implement safe techniques at work, it looks like in order to help decrease the stress load on his body while his back is recovering, the main modifications he needs to make have to do with some of his routine everyday activities. The main one for Ed is his sleeping position. The time he feels the most pain is during the middle of the night or first thing in the morning. He wakes up on his belly, lying face down, in a lot of pain, and trying to move out of that position is usually extremely painful for him.

When he is at work, up and about, he usually is able to move without too much pain at all because he is naturally very mindful of his mechanics and now pays extra attention to his forward leaning tasks in the kitchen and bathroom as well; he is careful to not be lazy and instead makes the effort to use his thighs and buttocks rather than locking his knees and letting his lower back round forward. It doesn't take much convincing to get Ed to agree to make the effort to avoid sleeping on his stomach. He explains that lying on his side is very comfortable and if he stays there he does not wake in pain. Sure enough, the relief he gets from his chiropractic treatments starts lasting longer each time, once he commits to avoiding the face-down sleeping position.

It seemed like this change in sleeping positions was the answer, but about one month after the initial episode, Ed developed another bout of the same pain—even worse this time. Although he had been doing a good job by not lying on his belly to sleep, this time when his pain came back, the previously helpful side-sleeping was really uncomfortable too. So, some fine-tuning of his back pain prevention strategy was needed. In Ed's case, this was because of a small change in his daily work routine.

There was a new work situation with Ed's latest project that had him occasionally standing, facing forward but reaching to the left. This work-related twist position was a new stressor for his already vulnerable lower back, and even though he did not notice pain at work, the result was evident in bed at night. Because of the additional and new work position stress, the tiny bit of additional twisting that happens when he lies on his side in bed at night and his top leg falls forward onto the mattress is no longer within tolerance and just reproduces the new twisting stress at work. It's a small deviation but still far enough outside of Ed's neutral mechanical "safe zone" (as dictated by his individual blueprint for optimal mechanical functioning[22]) that it registers as unacceptable during this delicate time in his recovery, while the fire of inflammation is still simmering, thereby creating less room for error during everyday life.

In Ed's case, this flare-up happened just a couple of weeks after his first bout with pain had started to feel better. The embers were still aglow and so it didn't take much to re-ignite everything. Together, while troubleshooting during one of his treatments, we found that now he would

---

22. Refer to Chapter 2 on page 34 for a reminder of the spine's optimal shape.

just need to add a pillow between his knees while lying on his side. This additional support between his legs is to keep his top leg from pulling his low back into a twist (causing shearing and lengthening stress[23]) as it falls forward onto the mattress.

Avoiding triggers is very important when you're trying to let your body recover from strain, but the best strategy I know of that will help you *completely avoid* recurrences of everyday pain once you've returned to a mostly pain-free life is to begin, as soon as possible, with a plan to buffer or bolster your body and lifestyle against future strain. You do this by eliminating as many mechanically stressful body positions or activities as you can, making this your new normal. The main purpose of this chapter is to help you identify what those stressful body positions or activities are. If you successfully teach yourself to avoid re-triggering your pain with innocent day-to-day activities, *then* you'll be ready to take the next step and start strengthening and reinforcing the area against those inevitable future occasions when certain triggers are briefly unavoidable.

The long term goal is to provide your body with a safety net and build up "money in the bank" to buy yourself time and tolerance. This sort of buffer will allow you to meet and stand up to all the different stressors that can accumulate day to day and put you at risk for setting off this pain again weeks, months or even years down the road. Once you know which of all three types of stressors are the ones *you* are most vulnerable to, you can target your fire-proofing approach as you prepare for the marathon of life with your particular physical, chemical and emotional machine of a body.

This third section of the book will guide you through the important task of discovering what your individual triggers are. We begin by considering *mechanical* triggers of strain and inflammation. First ask yourself these two things:

1. "What was I doing when the pain first hit?"
2. "What makes it hurt the most now?" ("In what position and with what activity?")

---

23. Refer to Chapter 2 on page 21 for additional information on mechanical triggers.

With this information, attention can then shift to discovering ways to lessen or avoid these triggering situations and find safe changes to the corresponding habits.

It's important to point out here that even if the situation, activity and position that you were in when you first felt pain was something you do all the time, please realize that it *still* must be avoided at all costs until you're out of pain again. Your body is not defective just because it suddenly didn't like that familiar situation. Even if it angers you and doesn't make *any* sense to you at all based on your past experience with your body, do not think you can demand from it, while it is in pain, to return to the situation that started the pain without experiencing significant consequences. Just like all those times you were able to do that thing without any pain at all, you might very well be able to do that thing without your current pain feeling too much worse—you may even get used to the pain and decide that it's not so bad after all. But take my word for it, you *are* just going to make things worse by not modifying your behavior.

The answers to "When does it hurt the most?" and: "What was I doing when the pain first hit?" will primarily shed light on your *mechanical* vulnerabilities. When it comes to your *chemical* and *emotional* weak spots, the discussion becomes a bit more generalized and perhaps even more thought provoking because of the wider array of possibilities, as we'll see in Chapter 8.

Once you've had some help identifying the pain triggers that you need to pay attention to, you'll be able to find an organized approach in the first chapter of the next volume on "Mechanical Repair" to help you create your own personalized buffers against a variety of common mechanical triggers. You'll find out how to reinforce against them with tools like specific isometric exercises, brain re-training and strengthening work. The goal is to not have to rely so heavily on always moving the *perfectly* safe way. Even though you will find that modifying your habits is an important part of the process to help you avoid re-injury, we all know that real life doesn't always allow us to behave "perfectly" 100% of the time. The long term and most realistic solution is going to be to make the best out of imperfect situations. So, we had better plan for those times when we need to cut corners, and the purpose of Volumes Two and Three (*Fix the Fire Damage* and *Plan For Fire Prevention* respectively) will be to show you how.

"Fire Proof" Body Mechanics

The most common trap for the average sufferer of these everyday injuries is the host of different things we do in order to just go about our daily routines. No matter how much of a he-man or she-woman athlete you think you are or actually have legitimately been at some point in your life, it's the basic little things you do every day to deal with the routine tasks of eating, sleeping, caring for your personal hygiene and earning a living that are actually the greatest and most common sources of aggravation to any kind of pain or injury you might be dealing with. Everything from sleeping positions or getting out of bed in the morning, to loading the dishwasher and driving to work, not to mention what you do while you're at work—all of it needs your serious attention for re-evaluation if you are going to put this everyday pain in its place. Keep it from coming back by developing and refining fire-proof mechanics. It's essential that you identify and avoid your main daily and repetitive triggers.

A not so funny age-old "joke" comes to mind here: a patient says to the doctor, "It hurts when I…" and the doctor replies brilliantly, "Well, then stop doing that!" What's amusing about that bad old joke is that while underlining the not-so-mystical insights of the physician, it isn't actually such far-fetched advice! Avoiding pain triggers is truly an important piece of information to take away from our experiences of pain. If it hurts to do A, B or C, then we have to respect that fact and find a way to avoid those things. It may only be temporary while the stressed area is allowed to recover—like the way a bandage would protect an open wound while it's healing—or it may be an opportunity to make some really smart modifications that will change how you move forever and for the better.

Possible Mechanical Triggers by Everyday Activity:

What follows is a rough visual list—a photographic guide—of the most common mechanical irritants that I encounter with my patients. During the course of

"The goal is to not have to rely so heavily on always moving the perfectly safe way."

treatment, these are the things that we have to address and re-work or learn to avoid, based on the location of our pain. If you apply the information from Chapter 2 about how the mechanics of the way we move and hold ourselves can be a recipe for trouble, you'll see that these are all examples of situations that place us in a sub-optimal position and force us to operate outside of our natural neutral zone.[24] I encourage you to come up with more such examples on your own that are specific to your situation and lifestyle.

If you are thinking to yourself: "Shouldn't I be able to do some of these ordinary and simple things without expecting to hurt myself (…insert expletive…)?" you are absolutely right. It's not wrong at all to expect to be able to do all of these things with ease and without pain, *but,* when we are injured and in pain, these are the things that will slow down and hinder recovery if they are not modified appropriately. The reality is that some of these activities, when done repetitively for a whole lifetime, are really only behaviors we get away with for so long because of the very forgiving nature of our un-injured, highly elastic body tissues. As soon as we experience strains and start forming protective adhesions (some of which just happens more easily as we age[25]), that elasticity of ours diminishes, and so does our ability to get away with all of the "bad" body behavior.[xlvii] Examples include inefficient movement patterns like reaching overhead instead of using a stepladder, or any prolonged strained positioning like falling asleep while reading in bed or on the couch.

The only reasonable way you can expect the human body to put up with these sub-optimal mechanical situations is to strengthen and reinforce your structure. (The first chapter of Volume Two will show you an organized approach to carefully start

---

24. Refer to Chapter 2 on page 34.

25. Be careful here! Don't let yourself get drawn into thinking that aging necessarily brings an increase in pain. The decrease in tissue elasticity is something we can influence in big ways through exercise and nutritional intake at every stage of our lives.

strengthening based on where it hurts.) With added muscle mass comes not only added strength but greater elasticity,[xlviii,xlix,l] and therefore, by extension, increased tolerance for imperfect situations. The main reason for the weak link that led to your pain is either a loss of physical conditioning or ongoing one-sided conditioning because of the often, one-sided demands of daily living.

The section that follows now in *this* chapter is designed to help you, at a glance, easily examine some common examples of activities in your everyday life that need to change in order to help keep your everyday pain at bay. You'll see these examples divided into 7 different types of situations common to everyday life:

1. Reaching
2. Reading and Writing
3. Sitting
4. Lying Down
5. Carrying
6. House and Yard
7. Self Care

Many of the images are of things that we all do without thinking twice until there's pain. I've tried to capture these common activities or situations with contrasting photographs: first to show you an example of when things can unexpectedly go wrong, then some suggestions for making the best of a potentially bad situation.

Some themes that you'll notice have to do with where your arms, head and torso are positioned in relationship to the body's "center". This refers to the center of gravity which is different for all of us but generally located somewhere behind the belly button. It's the point which grounds us in balance.

The closer you keep your body parts to that center of gravity, the less stress there is on all parts of the spine—the less work your body structures have to do to keep you from falling over (in theory). The farther away our limbs or head are from the torso center point, the greater the compressive force is on the spine. Compressive force exerted on the spine is calculated by multiplying distance away from center by the weight of the object and body part itself. This means that you can increase the amount of compression on your spine exponentially, simply by holding your arm out whether or not you have an object in your hand.

As you look over this section, keep in your mind's eye the idea of moving like a robot—as a protective strategy. You'll notice this often translates into keeping your *nose, toes and belly* pointing in the same direction as much as realistically possible during movement. Early classic robots are also only capable of forward and backward motion as elbows stay bent and close to the torso.

Another theme for executing movement safely during pain needs to be the concept of "neutral spine". Let me take you back to Figure 2.9 of Chapter 2 where I propose a rather socially counter-intuitive take on optimal spinal shape. It starts with a healthy active sway in the lower back and moves up into the mid and upper back with an equal yet opposite curling forward—almost hunching in contrast to military posture standards. Finally at the very top: a sway in the neck that mirrors the one in the low back but on a proportionately smaller scale—just enough to tip the chin up and allow an easy forward gaze. These curves have been vilified but they are the source of ease and relief for our struggling muscles during times of everyday pain crisis.

I encourage you to use this photographic guide to help identify other possible mechanical triggers specific to *your* day-to-day demands. I hope it gives you ideas about ways to re-think them for best results when trying to keep your own everyday pain from happening again. See if you can spot the three mechanical stressors in each scenario: compression, lengthening and shearing (twisting). Then think about where these stressors might be occurring for you.

Fire-Proof Body Mechanics

The Visual Guide

Prevent Reaching Pain in the Car

ARE YOU DOING THIS?

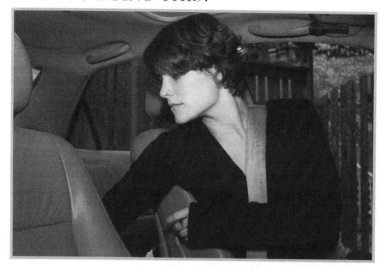

OR THIS?

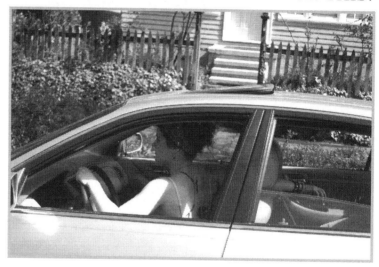

WHY IS THIS RISKY?

- Lower back is twisting = shearing stress
- Arm reach increases the compressive load on the entire spine
- Head leaning causes lengthening stress at the neck with twisting/ shearing stress

TRY THIS INSTEAD:

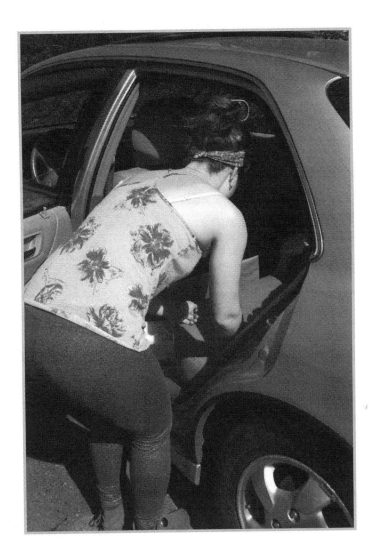

SAFER OPTION:

- Wait
- Get out of the car and reach into the back seat from the back door
- Knees together
- Buttocks out
- Neutral back as much as possible—allow the lower back sway

ARE YOU DOING THIS?

WHY IS THIS RISKY?

- Knees are locked
- Arms with object too far from center
- Back and neck are burdened with lengthening stress from the long reach

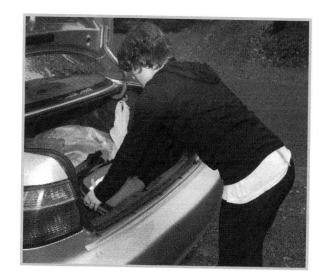

TRY THIS INSTEAD:

SAFER OPTION:

- Bend knees
- Move closer to the target
- Lean against bumper for added stability
- Decrease the distance between hands and center of gravity—shorter reach = less lengthening stress

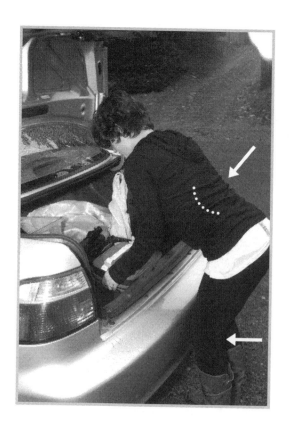

ARE YOU DOING THIS?

WHY IS THIS RISKY?

- One foot, both arms and head are far away from center of gravity
- Impact on spine is amplified compressive stress

TRY THIS INSTEAD:

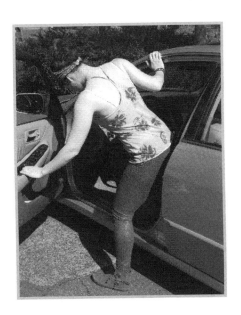

...THEN THIS

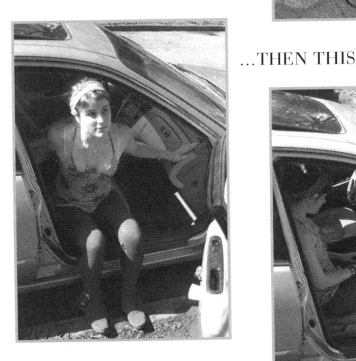

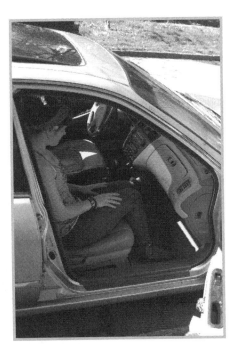

SAFER OPTION:

- Sit down first
- Swivel and lift one leg into the car at a time
- Keep limbs and torso as close to center as possible
- Avoid twisting and bending

Notice: Nose, toes and belly facing the same direction as much as possible during movement

Prevent Reaching Pain in the Kitchen

ARE YOU DOING THIS?

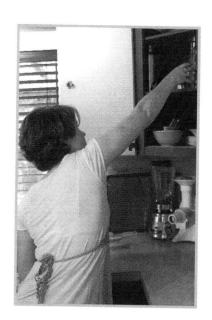

WHY IS THIS RISKY?

- The raised shoulder is maxed out and transferring extra work to the neck and back
- Hand is too far away from torso—triggers protective action in the back and side
- Side of the torso is being over-stretched creating lengthening stress

TAKE TIME TO DO THIS:

SAFER OPTION:

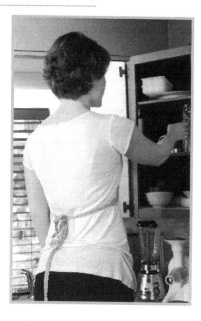 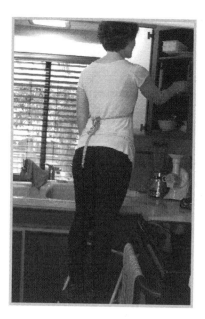

- Get a stepping stool and raise your center of gravity to decrease the reach
- Keep your elbows close to your torso
- Keep torso as upright as possible

ARE YOU DOING THIS?

WHAT'S RISKY ABOUT THIS?

- Belly is not facing the same direction as the object (pan) being reached for
- Hand is far away from center of gravity—multiplies compressive force on the spine
- Left lower back and left side of neck are being over-stretched causing lengthening stress

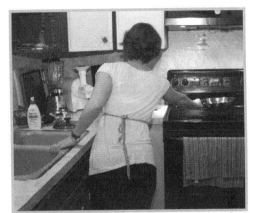

TRY THIS INSTEAD:

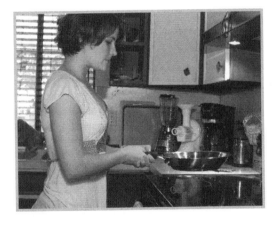

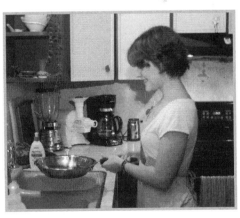

SAFER OPTION:

- Move your torso with your reach
- Fully face the object you're moving (toes, nose and belly point in the same direction)
- Keep elbows as close to torso as possible

ARE YOU DOING THIS?

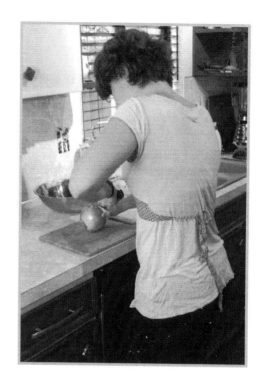

WHY IS THIS RISKY?

- Counter is too high, forcing shoulder and neck to strain
- Head and shoulder position are causing lengthening stress to neck and compressive stress to shoulder and upper back

TRY THIS INSTEAD:

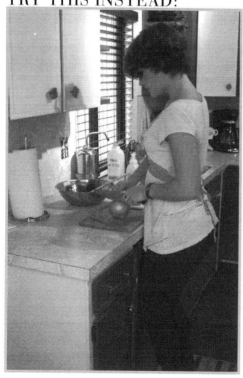

SAFER OPTION:

- Use a step/platform to stand on
- Allow power to be generated from lower core instead of shoulder and neck
- Bring elbow closer to torso

ARE YOU DOING THIS?

WHY IS THIS RISKY?

- Lower back and neck are rounding and reaching beyond neutral
- Knees are locked

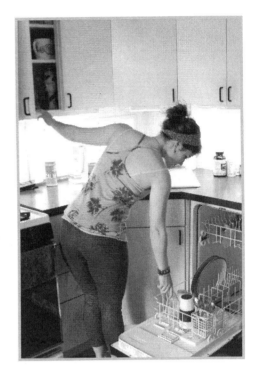

TRY THIS INSTEAD:

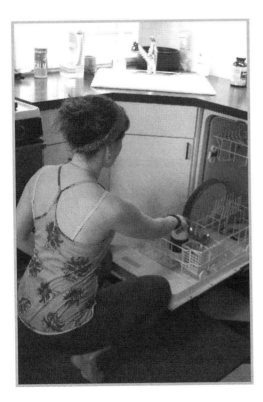

SAFER OPTION:

- Squatting or kneeling
- Bring center/belly closer to object
- Keep torso neutral

Prevent Reaching Pain in the Bathroom

ARE YOU DOING THIS?

WHY IS THIS RISKY?

- Knees are locked
- Hand is far away from belly
- Torso is leaning and rounding forward
- Head and chin are jutting forward
- Long reach is causing extra compression on spine

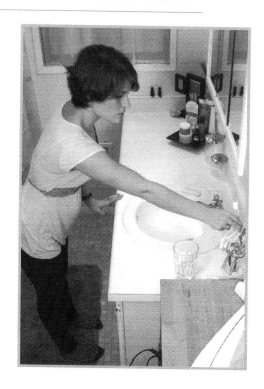

TRY THIS INSTEAD:

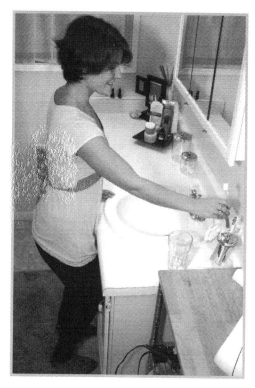

SAFER OPTION:

- Bend knees
- Lean legs against counter for support
- Keep torso as neutral as possible

ARE YOU DOING THIS?

WHY IS THIS RISKY?

- Knees are locked
- Back is rounding forward—lengthening and compressing
- Elbow is far from center
- Long reach by head and arm is multiplying compressive load on spine

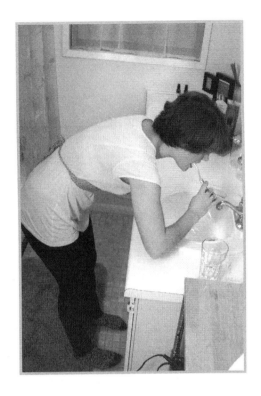

TRY THIS INSTEAD:

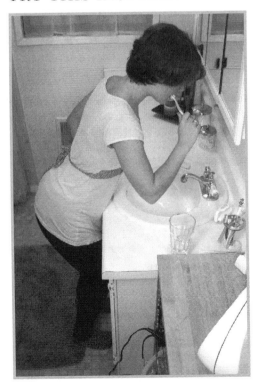

SAFER OPTION:

- Knees bent
- Thighs and knees leaning against counter for added support
- Relax the belly
- Let buttocks stick out
- Bring elbow in closer to torso

ARE YOU DOING THIS?

No Counter to lean your knees on?

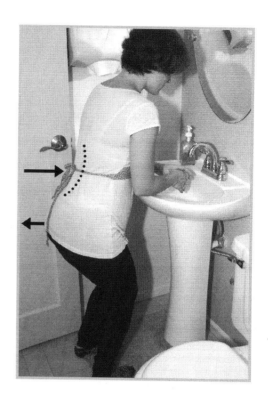

TRY THIS INSTEAD:

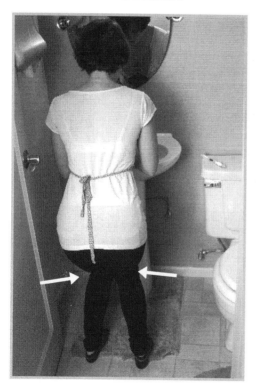

When there's lower back strain this can be helpful:

- Squeeze your knees together to create a tripod stabilization effect
- Buttocks out and belly relaxed

ARE YOU DOING THIS?

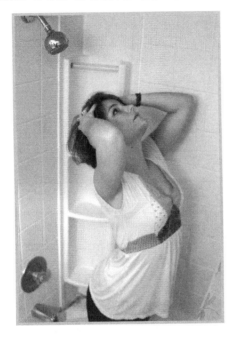 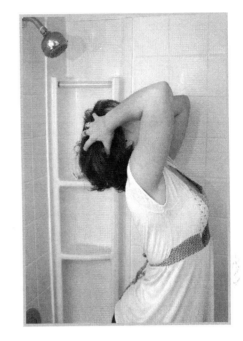

WHY IS THIS RISKY?

- Overarching lower back = compressive stress
- Overstretching front of neck = lengthening stress
- Arms over head adds imbalance and shoulder stress and transfers extra work to neck

TRY THIS INSTEAD:

SAFER OPTION:

- Unlock knees
- Squat
- Keep everything as close to center as possible

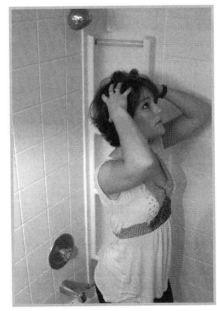

Prevent Reaching Pain in the Living Room

ARE YOU DOING THIS?

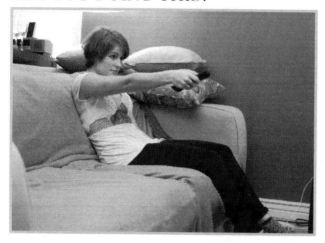

...OR THIS...

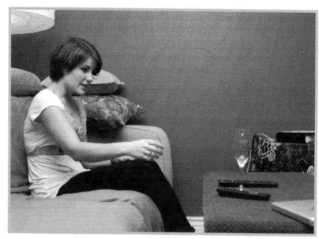

...OR THIS...?

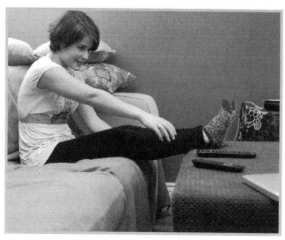

WHY IS THIS RISKY?

- Torso is curling
- Entire back and neck suffers lengthening stress
- Front of spine is suffering compression stress
- Reaching arm adds extra compressive stress to already stressed spine

STOP IT.

When there is back pain and inflammation, tucking the pelvis and tightening the abs during antics like these is *not at all* protective in already structurally risky situations.

Be careful: Just because you're strong in your core during workouts at the gym doesn't mean that abdominal bracing will help you get away with risky mechanics like this especially in an injured state. Abdominal bracing can actually amplify compressive stress for an injured back.

DO THIS INSTEAD:

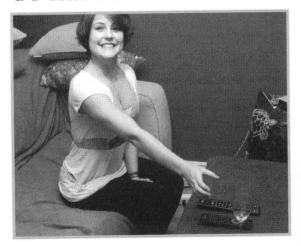

SAFER OPTION:

- Make the effort to bring your torso to neutral and scoot to the edge of the couch first

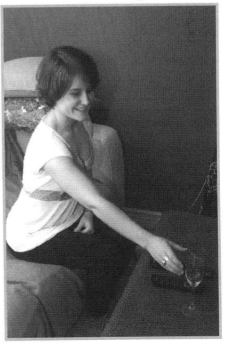

BETTER YET:

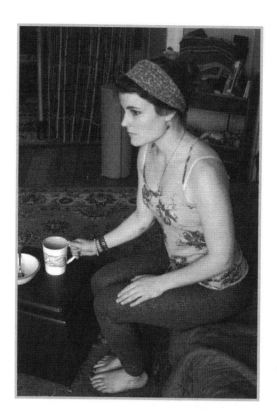

EVEN SAFER OPTION:

- Position yourself at the edge of your seat
- Keep torso neutral
- Knees together for added stability
- Elbows stay close to center

Prevent Reaching Pain in the Bedroom

ARE YOU DOING SOMETHING LIKE THIS?

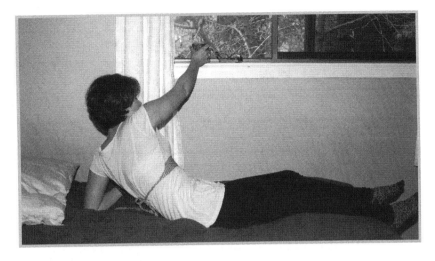

Making your abs and hip flexors work like this by sitting straight up from a resting position can trigger extreme protective guarding by the back muscles.

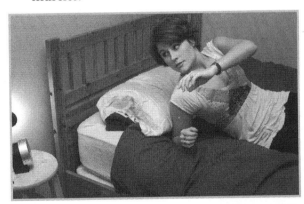

...OR ARE YOU DOING THIS (REACHING FOR THE ALARM)?

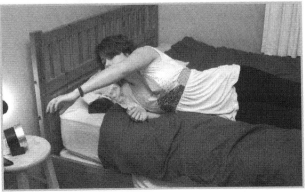

WHY ARE THESE SCENARIOS RISKY?

- Shearing stress
  - Lower back twisting
  - Mid-back twisting
- Lengthening stress
  - One-sided neck overstretch
  - One-sided torso overstretch
- Compressive stress
  - Weight-bearing shoulder joint
  - Reaching arm creates added load on neck and upper back

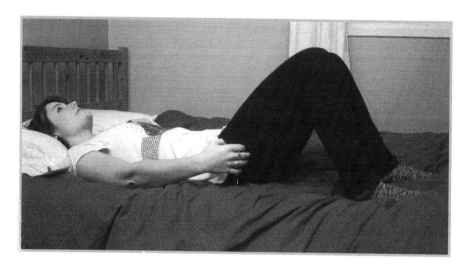

TAKE THE TIME TO GET UP SAFELY FIRST:

- Keep nose, toes and belly facing the same direction as much as possible throughout
- Bend knees
- Plant feet
- Squeeze buttocks and hold

TRY THIS NEXT:

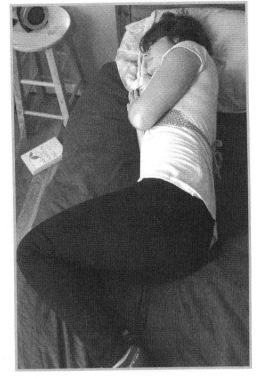

- Push up using your arms and elbows
- Find yourself facing the mattress as you push up
- Let feet drop off the edge and allow weight of legs to counterbalance and bring torso up
- Roll to side

THEN:

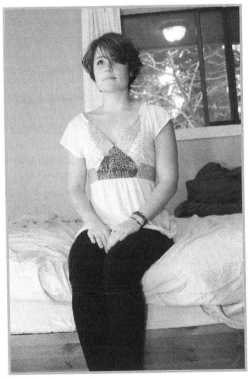

- Follow instructions on getting up safely from Chapter 5 page 97
- Once your safely upright reaching is much less risky
- Always keep your reach close to your torso center

Preventing Reading and Writing Pain at the Desk

ARE YOU DOING THIS WITH YOUR BOOK OR E-READER?

WHY IS THIS RISKY?

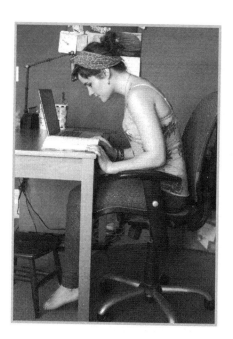

- Forward head reach is multiplying compression on spine of the lower and mid-back
- Rounding spine is contributing to lengthening stress on neck, mid-back and lower back
- Feet are unsupported—causing silent activation of hip flexors (e.g., iliopsoas, quadriceps) where the torso joins with the legs in the front

TRY THIS INSTEAD:

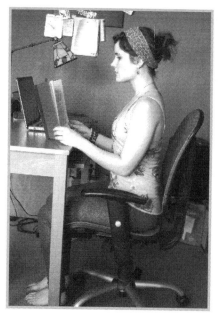

SAFER OPTION:

- Lower the seat to let feet rest on ground
- Let eyes gaze downward as long as chin can stay up
- Prop or hold book or e-reader up

ARE YOU DOING THIS WITH YOUR LAPTOP?

WHY IS THIS RISKY?

- Lengthening stress to:
    - Neck—upper back connection
    - Upper back
    - Lower back
- Compression stress made worse by:
    - Flat/rounded lower back
    - Long arm reach
    - Craning neck compresses neck-head connection

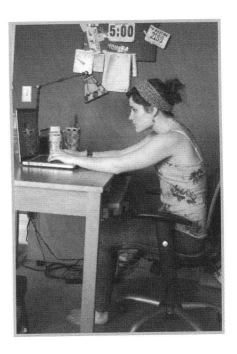

SOME SAFER OPTIONS:

- Wireless keyboard—alleviates arm reach with a laptop
- Raise chair and use foot rest
- Raise laptop to bring screen to eye level—keep gaze up and into the horizon

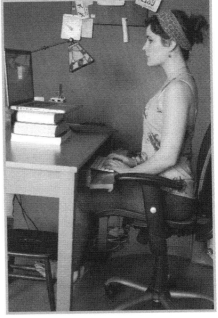

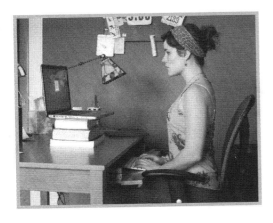

Preventing Reading and Writing Pain on the Couch

DO YOU DO THIS WITH YOUR LAPTOP?

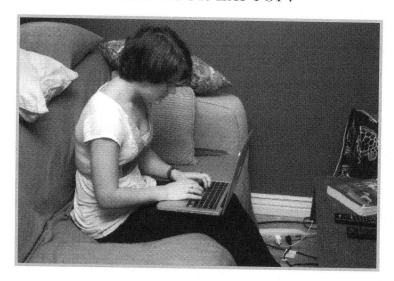

WHY IS THIS RISKY?

Back rounding and head reach causes both lengthening stress and compressive stress to neck, mid back and lower back.

TRY THIS:

SAFER OPTIONS:

- Let head rest back
- Use support in the small of the back
- Place laptop on a raised surface (cushion)
- Make sure feet are supported, legs are not dangling

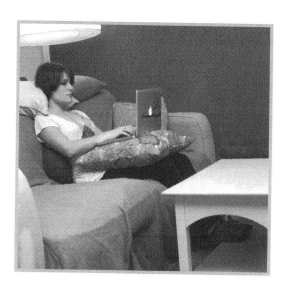

OR THIS:

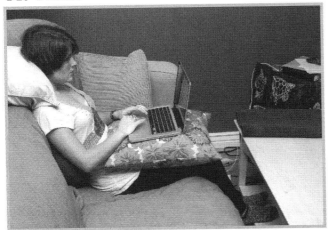

OR THIS:

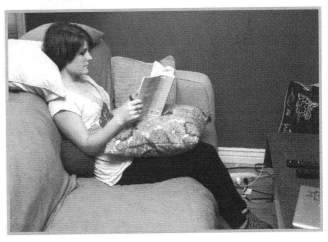

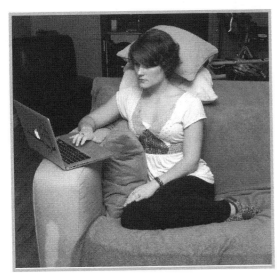

ALTERNATIVE OPTION:

- Acceptable only for *some* lower backs that are especially sensitive to compression *and* have the benefit of moderately flexible hips and legs
- This is an option but not ideal and especially not for extended periods of time

Preventing Reading and Writing Pain in the Bedroom

ARE YOU READING IN BED LIKE THIS?

WHY COULD THIS BE RISKY?

- Shoulder is being compressed
- Neck experiences lengthening stress on one side and compressive stress on the other
- Curled torso position causes compression stress in the front and lengthening stress in the back…although this is less severe when lying down and more so when sitting or standing

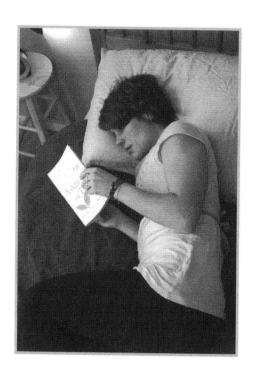

TRY THIS IMPERFECT COMPROMISE:

SOMEWHAT SAFER OPTIONS:

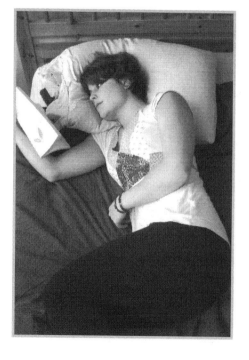

- Open the chest to decrease compression
- Lie on the flat part of the shoulder blade instead of directly on the arm
- Bring head and neck back
- Raise gaze and reading material

ARE YOU READING IN BED LIKE THIS?

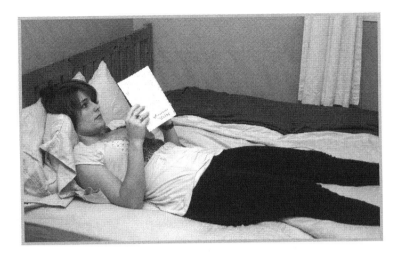

WHY IS THIS RISKY?

- Overstretch to the back of the neck causes lengthening stress at neck to shoulder blade connection compressive stress to the front of the neck at neck-chest connection
- Lower back rounding with variable support depending on the mattress—causes subtle compression in front of spine and subtle lengthening in lower back

TRY THIS INSTEAD:

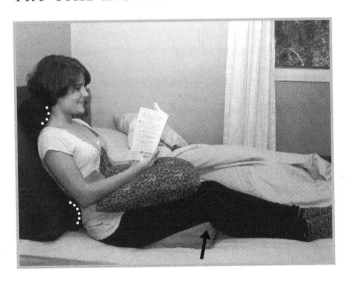

SAFER OPTION:

- Strive for neutral spine to allow muscles of neck, back and legs to rest and become slack

TRY THIS ONLY IF YOU DO NOT HAVE LOWER BACK PAIN:

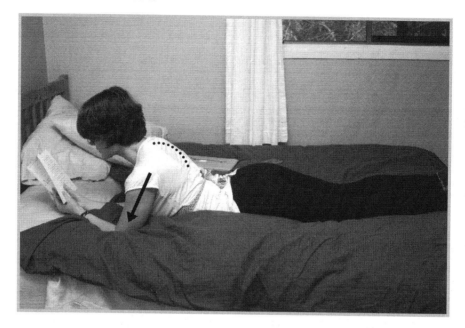

- Alternative for short-term positioning only
- In favor of productive neck and upper back activation
- Push with arms purposefully into the mattress to create and active, protective upper back and shoulder stance

ARE YOU DOING HOMEWORK ON THE FLOOR?

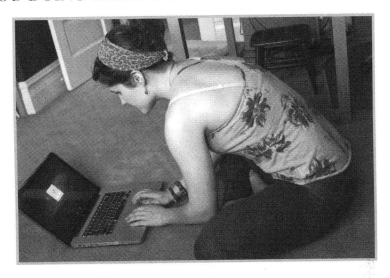

WHY IS THIS RISKY?

The tighter your legs, the more the lower back suffers in this situation due to lengthening and compressive stress from excessive rounding.

STILL NOT IDEAL, BUT TRY SOMETHING MORE LIKE THIS:

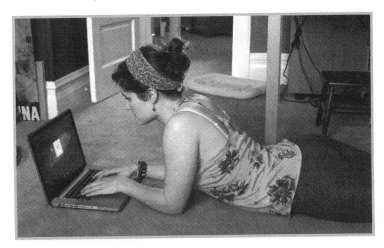

- For some, this *may* be a better option
- Still not ideal and not for long periods of time
- Approaches the neutral spine shape better than previous option

DO YOU WORK ON YOUR LAPTOP IN BED LIKE THIS?

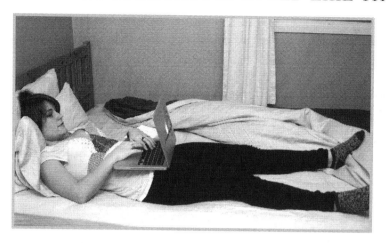

WHY IS THIS RISKY?

- Overstretch lengthening stress to back of neck-head and back of neck-shoulder connections
- Compressive stress to front of neck and neck-chest connection

THINK ABOUT TRYING THIS:

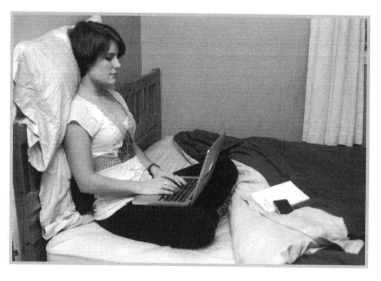

SAFER OPTION:

- Strive for neutral spine, which allows muscles to relax

IF YOU CAN'T SIT WITH LEGS IN LOTUS POSITION, TAKE THE TIME TO DO THIS...

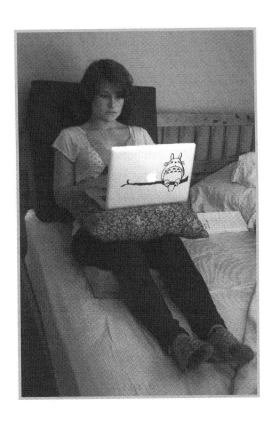

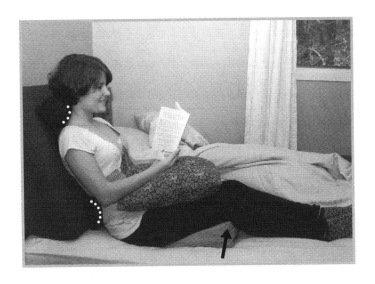

Preventing Sitting Pain While Dining

ARE YOU DOING THIS?

WHY IS THIS RISKY?

- Compressive stress to the lower back
- Forward head reach multiplies this compression
- Lengthening stress to mid-back and neck

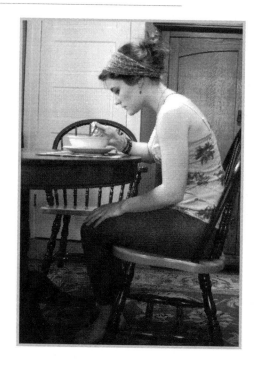

TRY THIS INSTEAD:

SAFER OPTION:

- Decrease head reach and arm reach
- Bring food to mouth, not mouth to food

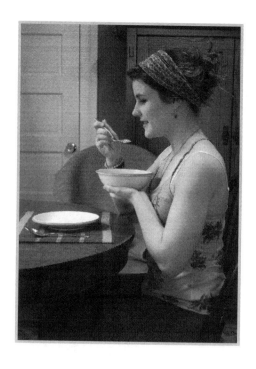

ARE YOU EATING AT THE COUCH IN FRONT OF THE TV?

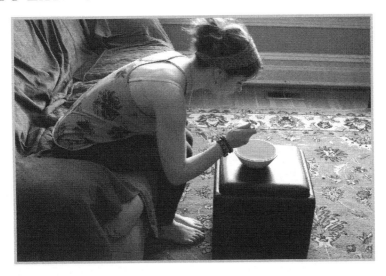

WHY IS THIS RISKY?

- Compressive stress to the lower back
- Forward head reach multiplies this compression
- Lengthening stress to mid-back and neck

DO YOUR BEST TO SIMULATE THIS:

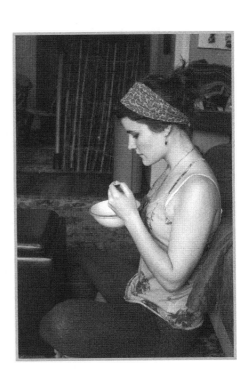

SAFER OPTION:

- Decrease head reach and arm reach
- Bring food to mouth, not mouth to food

Preventing Sitting Pain on the Couch
(Watching TV)

ARE YOU DOING THIS?

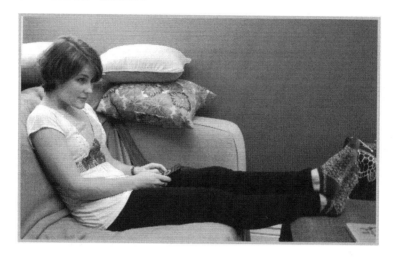

WHY IS THIS RISKY?

- Head is migrating forward center causing lengthening and compressive stresses
- Lower back rounding with head drift causes amplified compressive and lengthening stress

THIS IS BETTER FOR SOME:

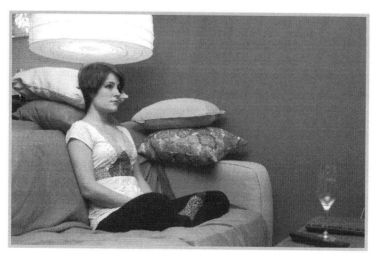

THIS CAN BE BETTER FOR OTHERS:

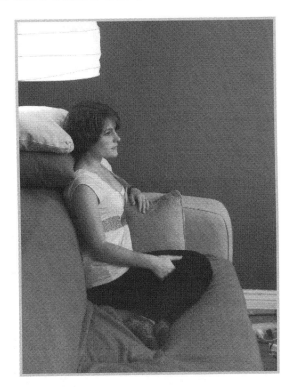

REMEMBER THIS?

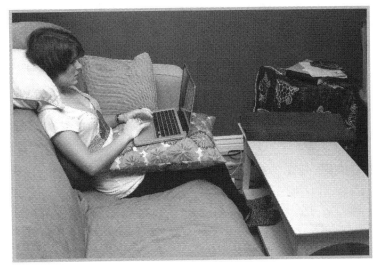

It works for watching TV, too.

Preventing Sitting Pain in Bed

ARE YOU DOING THIS?

This looks like a good effort, so…

WHY IS THIS RISKY?

- Head is pitched forward
- Entire spine is C-shaped despite the nice pillow set-up, which causes lengthening and compression stress up and down the spine

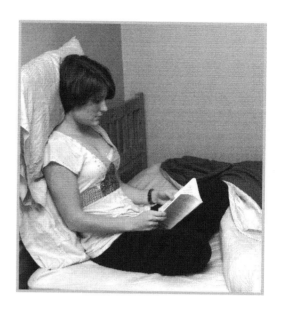

THINK ABOUT TRYING THIS:

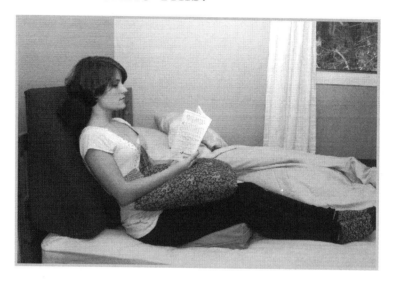

SAFER OPTION:

- Support knee bend
- Support small of back gentle sway
- Rest head back
- Support neck sway

Preventing Sitting Pain at Work

ARE YOU DOING THIS?

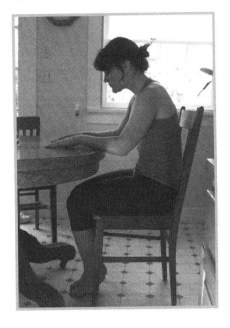

THINK ABOUT TRYING THIS:

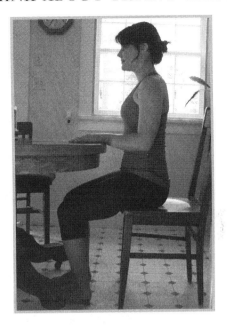

Preventing Sitting Pain in the Car

ARE YOU DOING THIS?

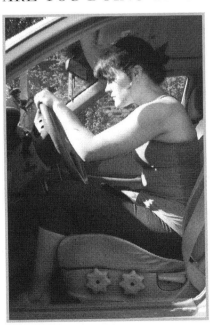

THINK ABOUT TRYING THIS:

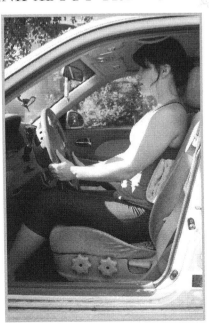

Preventing Pain While Lying on Your Side

ARE YOU DOING THIS?

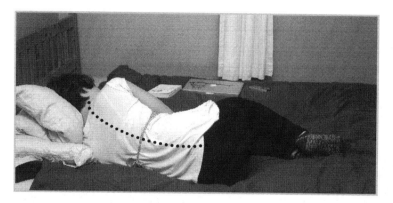

WHY IS THIS RISKY?

- Head too high
- Lengthening stress on left side of neck-shoulder connection
- Subtle shearing stress from twisting between lower and mid-back
- Slight left-sided lower back lengthening stress from waist droop into the mattress

TRY TO ACHIEVE THIS:

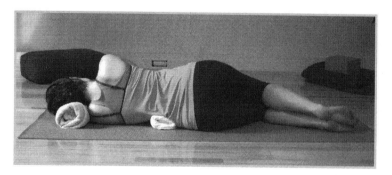

SAFER OPTIONS:

- Lower head and neck support to help you approach the neutral spine
- Add support at the waist
- Pillow between knees to prevent twisting (not pictured here)

WHICH MIGHT LOOK MORE LIKE THIS:

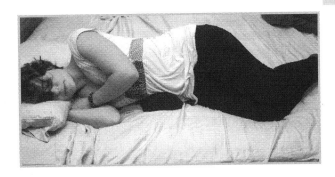

THIS CAN BE A GOOD OPTION, TOO:

NEUTRAL SPINE:

- All facing in the same direction:
  - Nose
  - Knees
  - Belly
- Keep arm close to torso
- Elbow below shoulder

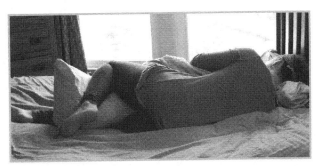

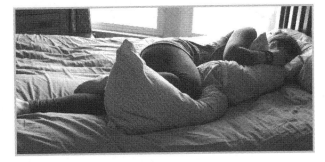

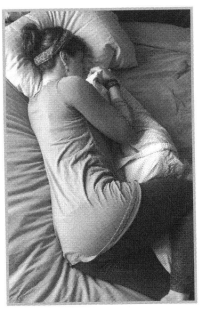

SAFE FEATURE:

- Close to neutral spine
- Support under top leg

IS THIS YOU ON THE COUCH?

ARE YOU DOING THIS?

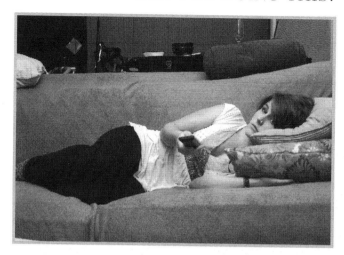

RISKY FEATURE:

Head elevated—
causing overstretched
lengthening stress
to shoulder-neck
connection

THIS IS BETTER, BUT BE CAREFUL OF THE TWISTING:

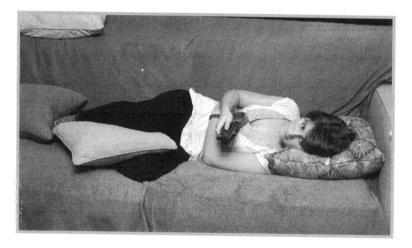

RISKY FEATURE:

- Shearing stress between mid and lower spine

SAFER FEATURE:

- Head more centered

THIS IS GOOD, BUT BE CAREFUL OF THE REACHING:

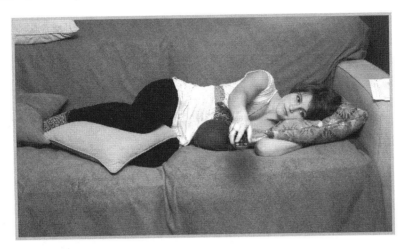

RISKY FEATURE:

- Reaching arm
- Compressed shoulder

SAFER FEATURE:

- Centered spinal alignment
- No shearing stress—no twist

Preventing Pain While Lying Face Up

ARE YOU DOING THIS?

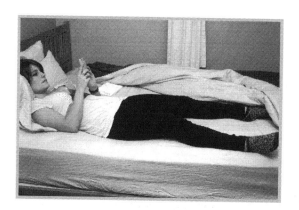

WHY IS THIS RISKY?

- Compressive stress to:
  - Front of the neck
  - Chest
  - Front of the lower spine

- Lengthening overstretch stress to:
  - Back of the neck-head connection
  - Neck-upper back connection
  - Neck-both shoulder blade connection

TRY TO ACHIEVE THIS:

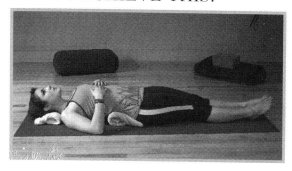

OR THIS:

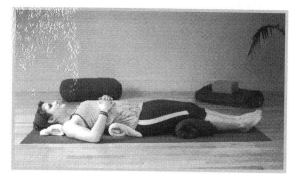

SAFER OPTIONS:

- Lie flat and put down the device
- Add support for a neutral spine:
  - Under the neck
  - Under the lower back/waist
  - Under the knees

Preventing Pain While Lying Face Down

DO YOU SOMETIMES DO THIS?

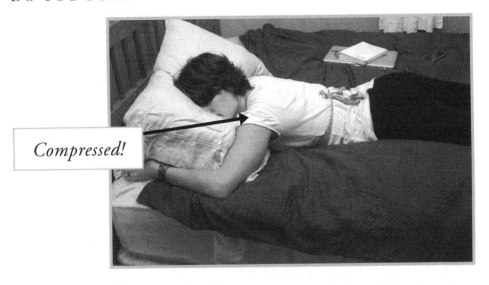

Compressed!

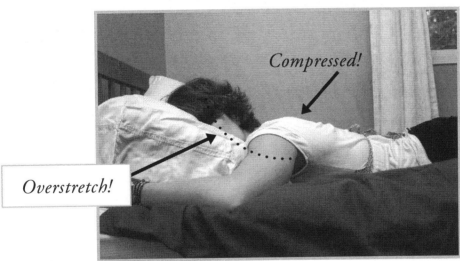

Compressed!

Overstretch!

WHY IS THIS RISKY?

- Head is too high
- Low back and back of neck are compressed
- Arm is too far up, causing compression at shoulder-neck connection

DID YOU KNOW THIS COULD BE AN "OKAY" COMPROMISE?

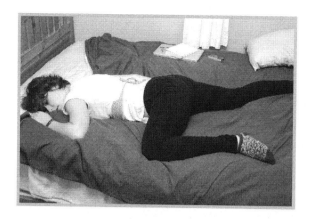

- All on the same side:
  - Head turn
  - Arm raised
  - Leg raised

SAFER OPTION:

- Only for those who are unable *not* to sleep face-down
- This is not for everyone!

...IF YOU MAKE SURE TO DO THIS:

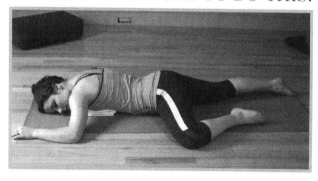

- Support under chest only
- No pillow under head!
- This will give you more of a neutral spine

...AND THIS:

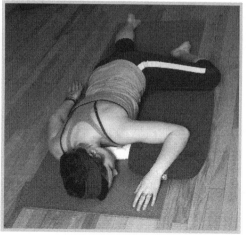

- Support under raised knee and raised arm to decrease twisting/ shearing stress
- Notice that elbow of raised arm does not go higher than shoulder level
- Very important!
  - Opposite arm must be down at side of torso
  - Front of shoulder flat against bed

Preventing Pain While Carrying Bags

DO YOU DO THIS WITH YOUR SPORTS BAG?

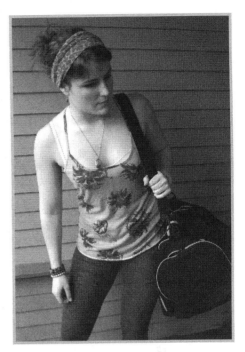

WHY IS THIS RISKY?

- Long strap throws off center of gravity pitching torso to one side
- Weight of bag rests between shoulder and hip—long reach creates pendulum effect that is difficult to control

TRY THIS INSTEAD:

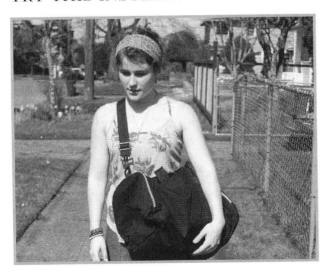

SAFER OPTION:

- Shorten strap
- Tuck and hug bag under arm and closer to torso

ARE YOU DOING THIS WITH YOUR BACK PACK?

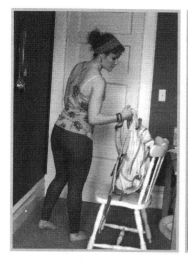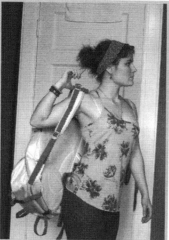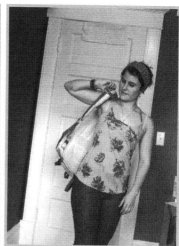

WHY IS THIS RISKY?

- One arm swing creates off-center compression, lengthening and shearing/twisting stress in numerous places
- Lifting weight from low to high through multiple planes of movement

TAKE TIME TO DO THIS INSTEAD:

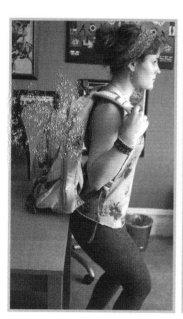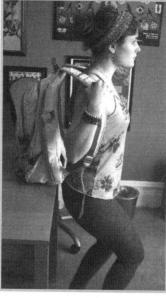

SAFER OPTION:

- "Step into" backpack straps
- Place bag on higher surface
- Use legs to squat to get into the straps
- Keep torso neutral and upright

ARE YOU DOING THIS WITH YOUR PURSE?

WHY IS THIS RISKY?

- Even without a lot of weight in the purse, the strap will reflexively trigger shoulder rise
- Lengthening stress to opposite neck-shoulder connection
- Compressive stress on the purse strap side neck-shoulder connection

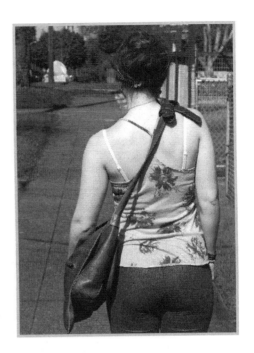

TRY THIS INSTEAD:

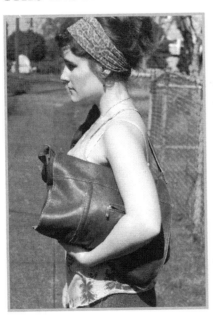

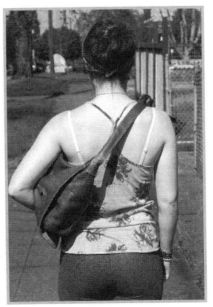

SAFER OPTION:

- Shorten strap
- Hug purse close to body
- Under arm or to chest

Preventing Pain Around the House and Yard

ARE YOU DOING THINGS LIKE THIS WHILE TIDYING OR CLEANING?

WHY IS THIS RISKY?

- Arms above shoulder height— transfers work to neck
- Looking up—compressive stress to neck and shoulders
- Distance between task and stable point (feet) too far
- Reach causes lengthening stress between shoulders, mid-back and low back

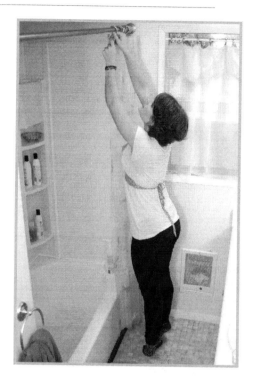

TAKE THE TIME TO DO THIS INSTEAD:

SAFER OPTION:

- Keep elbows at or below shoulder level
- Raise stance with a stepladder—get closer to your task

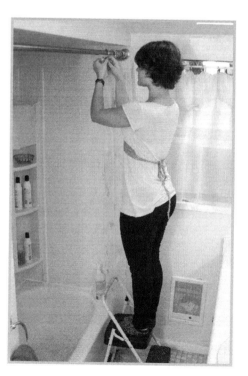

ARE YOU VACUUMING LIKE THIS?

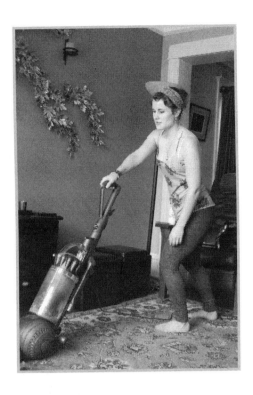

WHY IS THIS RISKY?

- Toes, nose and belly are not facing the same direction causing shearing stress via torso twist
- Arm reach
    - Multiplies compressive stress to low back
    - Causes lengthening stress to upper back

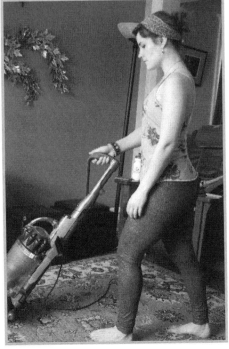

TRY THIS INSTEAD:

SAFER OPTION:

- Lunge stance
- Hold vacuum with opposite arm/hand from leading leg
- Hinge at hips and buttocks while lunging for forward backward motion
- Keep torso neutral

ARE YOU RAKING OR SWEEPING LIKE THIS?

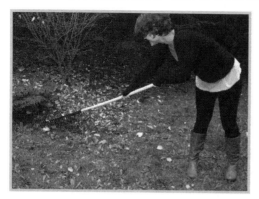 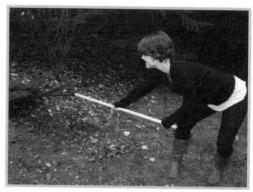

WHY IS THIS RISKY?

- Toes, nose and belly are not lined up—back is rounded and twisting
- Reaching arms and head amplify compression on spine
- Neck is alternately lengthened and compressed

TRY SOMETHING MORE LIKE THIS:

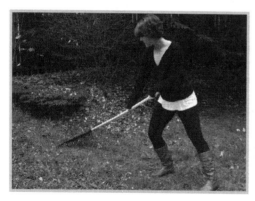 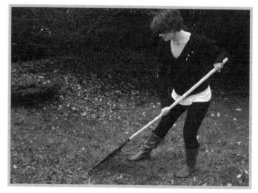

NOT PERFECT BUT SAFER OPTION:

- Line up nose, toes and belly as much as realistically possible
- Keep arm reach to a minimum
- Use lunging and squatting motion at hips and legs to achieve back-and-forth movements—not the lower back

IS THIS HOW YOU'RE DOING YOUR WEEDING?

WHY IS THIS RISKY?

- Seems like a good stretch? Don't do it!
- Low back rounding over-stretched and compressed
- Neck compressed
- Overstretched lengthening stress between shoulder and hips from arm reach as well as rounding

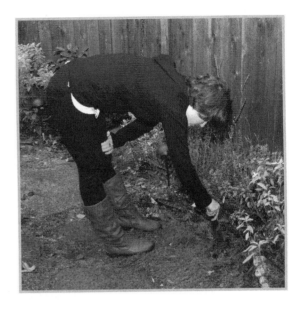

THIS IS BETTER:

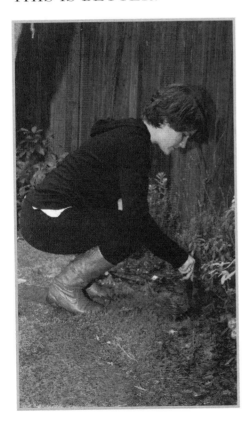

NOT PERFECT, BUT SAFER OPTION:

- Squat if legs will allow with neutral lower back
- If legs are too tight, this too will cause rounding and thereby compressive and lengthening low back stress
- For the flexible legs this is an "okay" way to decrease reach and minimize stress to back and neck
- Bring gardening task closer to body center

BUT THIS IS BETTER STILL:

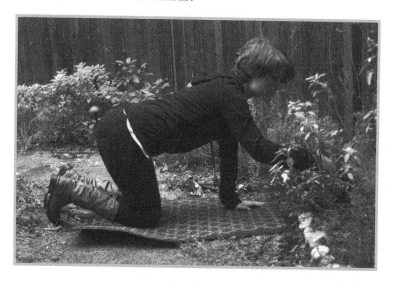

SAFER OPTION—STILL NOT PERFECT:

- Relief from gravity related compression to spine by taking horizontal position
- Keep neck and low back neutral—relax belly/un-tuck stick buttocks out
- Keep arm reach to a minimum
- Rich padding under knees
- Take breaks!

ARE YOU DOING THIS WHEN YOU'RE PRUNING?

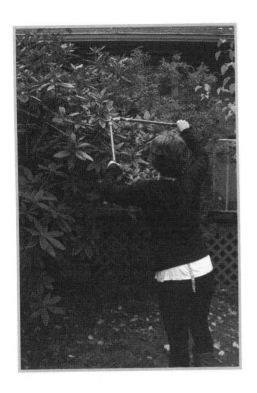

WHY IS THIS RISKY?

- Arms above shoulder height—transfers work to neck
- Looking up—compressive stress to neck and shoulders
- Distance between task and stable point (feet) too far
- Reach causes lengthening stress between shoulders, mid-back and low back

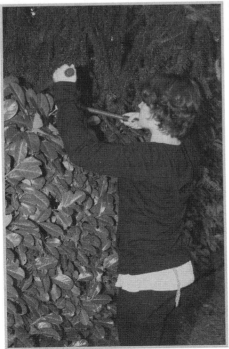

TAKE THE TIME TO DO THIS WHENEVER POSSIBLE:

SAFER OPTION:

- Keep elbows at or below shoulder level
- Raise stance with a stepladder—get closer to your task

ARE YOU DOING THIS WITH THE MOWER?

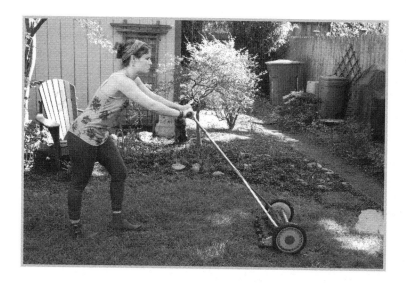

WHY IS THIS RISKY?

- Watch the reach:
  - Distance between target task and core is too great
- Arms off center—to the side
- Creates:
  - Shearing stress at torso
  - Compressive stress on one side
  - Lengthening stress to opposite side

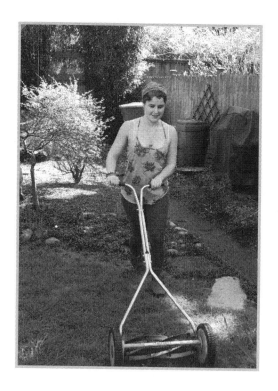

ALWAYS TRY FOR SOMETHING MORE LIKE THIS:

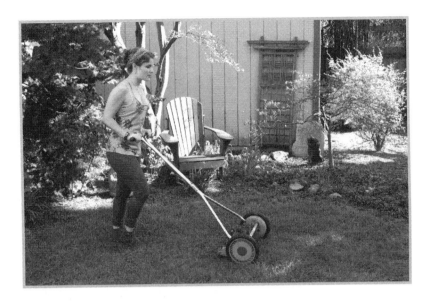

SAFER OPTION:

- Keep handle close to center
- Torso upright—no reaching
- Generate power from legs and center of gravity
- Move only one direction at a time:
  - Forward-backward
  - No sideways turning

Preventing Pain While Dressing and Washing

DO YOU PUT PANTS ON LIKE THIS?

<u>WHY IS THIS RISKY?</u>

- Unstable—recruits more muscle work than necessary
- Rounding spine
  - Compression
  - Lengthening
- Reaching is too far from forward from center

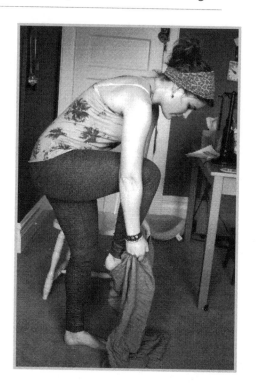

WHEN YOU'RE IN PAIN, TRY THIS:

<u>SAFER OPTION:</u>

- More stable
- Less rounding is possible but requires effort
- Less reaching

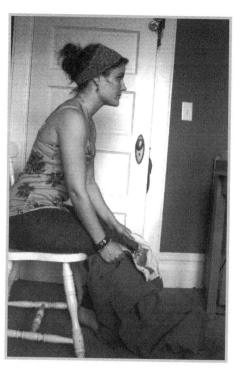

WORST-CASE SCENARIO, THIS MAY BE YOUR BEST BET:

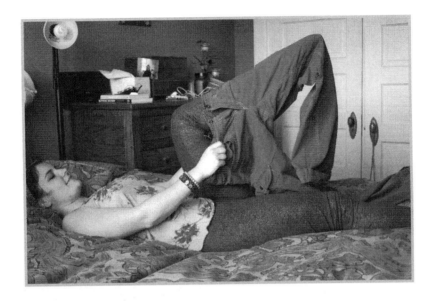

- Entire spine is supported here
- Lifting leg is now not as compressive to the spine as it is in the upright position with gravity to fight

DO YOU PUT YOUR SHOES ON LIKE THIS?

WHY IS THIS RISKY?

- Rounding causes lengthening stress
- Shearing stress from the side-to-side reach—subtle twist in torso and hips

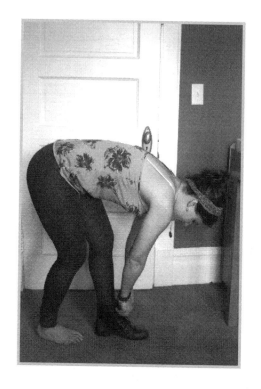

THIS MIGHT BE BETTER, BUT STILL NOT THE BEST:

SAFER OPTION WITH COMPROMISE:

- Sitting
  - Very compressive
  - Less rounding overstretch in low back
  - More rounding overstretch in upper back
- Shorter reach is better
- Hip stress
  - Stiffness may not allow for this option

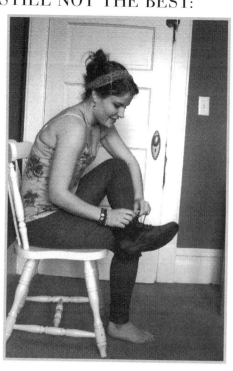

SOME PEOPLE MANAGE BY DOING THIS:

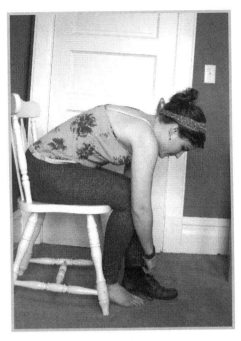

SAFER OPTIONS WITH COMPROMISES #2 & 3:

- Keep neutral spine by maintaining gentle sway in low back
- Still risky rounding and reaching
- Need hip and leg flexibility for these variations

THIS IS HOW TO MAKE THE BEST OF A BAD SITUATION:

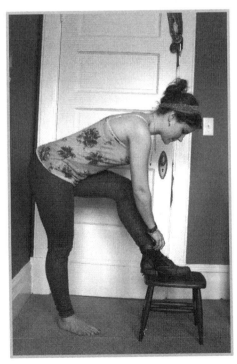

UNTIL YOUR PAIN PASSES, DO THIS:

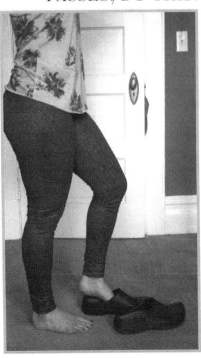

SAFEST OPTION:

- Give up laces until you feel better

IS THIS HOW YOU PUT YOUR JACKETS AND DRESS SHIRTS ON?

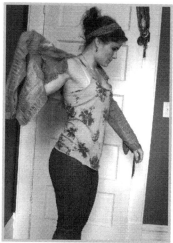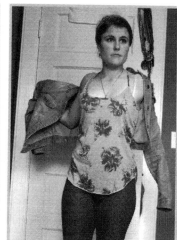

WHY IS THIS RISKY?

- Backward arm reach causes torso twisting = shearing stress on the spine
- Lengthening stress is also imposed on neck

THINK ABOUT TRYING THIS INSTEAD:

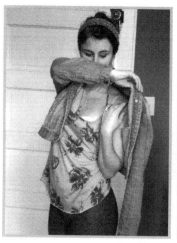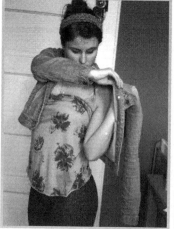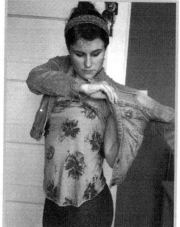

SAFER OPTION:

- One arm at a time
- Bring sleeve opening to shoulder instead of reaching with arm

DO YOU FIND YOURSELF DOING THIS TO GET INTO YOUR PULLOVERS?

WHY IS THIS RISKY?

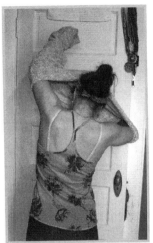

- Arms above shoulder and head—amplifies compressive stress to upper back and neck

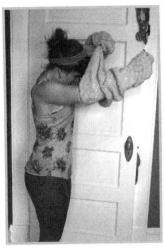

- Head reach creates lengthening stress to back of neck-head connection
- Arm position causes lengthening stress between shoulder blades and mid-low back area

THINK ABOUT TRYING THIS INSTEAD:

SAFER OPTION:

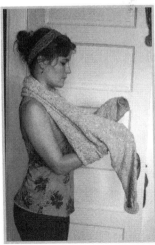

- Break it down:
  - Slip head through first
  - One arm at a time
  - Minimize reaching

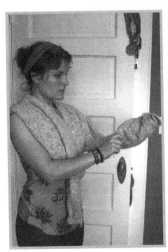

HOW DO YOU GET OUT OF YOUR PULLOVER SHIRTS?

WHY IS THIS RISKY?

- Raised arm crossover causes:
    - Compression in chest
    - Lengthening stress between shoulder blades
    - Arms over head amplifies compressive stress to entire spine

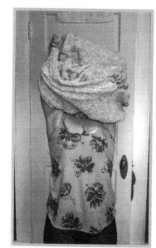
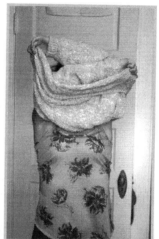

TRY THIS INSTEAD:

SAFER OPTION:

- Break it down:
    - Slide out of one sleeve at a time
    - Pull head out last

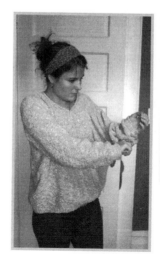
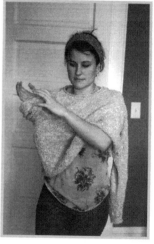

DO YOU DO THIS TO DRY, BRUSH OR STYLE YOUR HAIR?

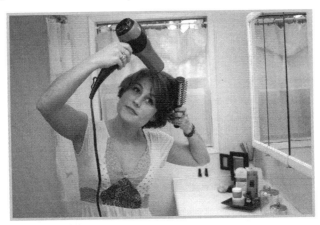

WHY IS THIS RISKY?

- Prolonged raised arms above shoulder level causes:
  - Compressive stress in neck and upper back
  - Arm fatigue leads to extra neck muscle recruitment

WHEN YOU'RE IN PAIN, GIVE THIS A TRY:

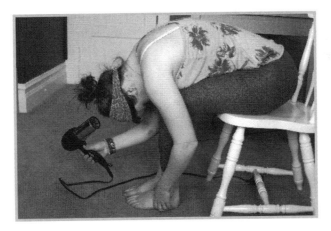

IMPERFECT ALTERNATIVE:

- Muscles are resting better
- Still requires care
- Rounding may not be optimal
- Hairstyle WILL suffer

DO YOU DO THIS WHILE YOU BRUSH YOUR TEETH?

WHY IS THIS RISKY?

- Knees are locked
- Back is rounding forward—lengthening and compressing
- Elbow is far from center
- Long reach by head and arm is multiplying compressive load on spine

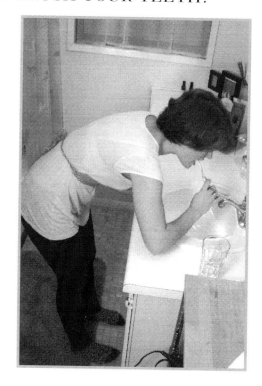

TRY THIS INSTEAD:

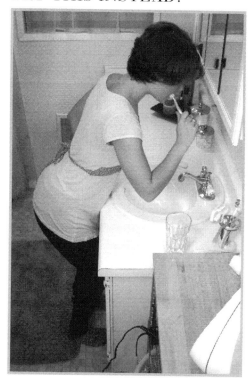

SAFER OPTION:

- Knees bent
- Thighs and knees leaning against counter for added support
- Relax the belly
- Let buttocks stick out
- Bring elbow in closer to torso

NO COUNTER TO LEAN YOUR KNEES ON? TRY THIS:

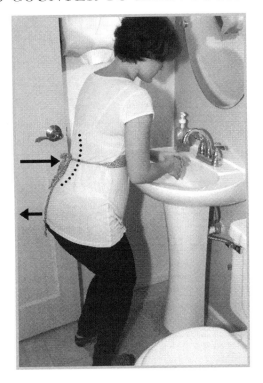

WHEN THERE'S LOWER BACK STRAIN THIS CAN BE HELPFUL:

- Squeeze your knees together to create a tripod stabilization effect
- Buttocks out and belly relaxed

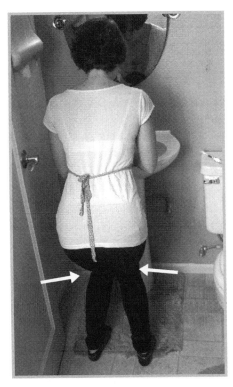

IS THIS HOW YOU WASH YOUR HAIR IN THE SHOWER?

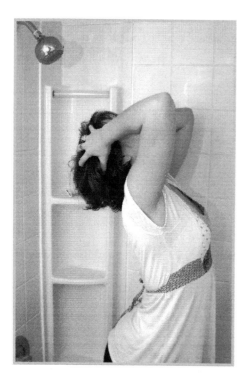

WHY IS THIS RISKY?

- Overarching lower back = compressive stress
- Overstretching front of neck = lengthening stress
- Arms over head add imbalance and shoulder stress and transfer extra work to neck

TRY SOMETHING MORE LIKE THIS:

SAFER OPTION:

- Unlock knees
- Squat
- Keep everything as close to center as possible

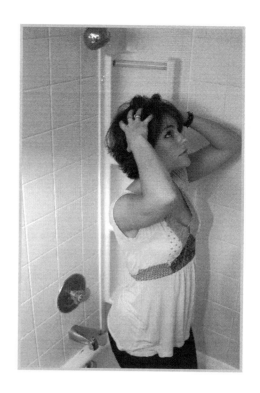

Final Reminders:

- Don't let yourself become preoccupied with feelings of embarrassment or defectiveness and self judgment. You are not alone.

- Many of these modifications might feel awkward and unfamiliar compared with what were previously "natural" habits, but remember that these are legitimate methods that will help speed your recovery.

- Even if you still feel your pain while faithfully implementing the safer movement options, you can rest assured that you are doing your part in preventing the situation from worsening. Most importantly, this means you don't have to be afraid to move.

CHAPTER 8

Fire Proof Body Chemistry

THE TWO QUESTIONS OF "WHEN DOES it hurt the most?" and "What was I doing when the pain first hit?" are definitely more oriented to the mechanical or structural groups of triggers. Now, when exploring your own unique *chemical* vulnerabilities, the better questions to ask yourself are:

1. *"Where* am I feeling the pain (and therefore inflammation)?"
2. *"What else* might be inflamed *nearby?"*

Sometimes the answer to this latter question should come from your doctor and with the help of some further testing and clinical investigating. But there's no reason you can't feed your healthy curiosity about neighboring structures and organs and how they may play a role in everyday pain at a subclinical[26] level—a level of dysfunc-

---

26. The term "subclinical" is used to denote conditions that do not present frank pathology or disease as recognized by the allopathic medical community. Instead, subclinical conditions can be suboptimal functioning resulting from systems out of balance, possibly a precursor to disease states.

tion or imbalance that is often not seen as "clinically significant" by mainstream medicine because there is no full blown disease process at this stage.

Please let me remind you that this book is only looking at everyday pain—not any of the more serious conditions or diseases that would require medical intervention. As we start to examine the multiple layers of chemical stressors/chemical triggers of pain, I welcome you to engage in a healthy dose of critical thinking, because, occasionally, I will be speaking from my experience in practice rather than necessarily referring to a solid body of research. Often, time-tested wisdom stands alone for decades, maybe centuries, before we can produce the kind of double-blinded evidence that is required of modern research to prove or validate what generations of non-mainstream practitioners have known and seen in action throughout the ages.

Keep in mind the groundwork of understanding about inflammation that was covered in Sections I and II and how it can be happening without our awareness and how it can spill over into neighboring areas. Now consider the fact that many internal structures and organs that your skeleton houses can experience bouts of inflammation for reasons unrelated to any mechanical factors. These bouts of inflammation (from non-mechanical sources) can occur without any big display of symptoms either, and, in fact, would be considered "subclinical" because there is no actual pathology or disease associated with these sorts of inflammatory spells.

As we saw in Chapter 3, chemical triggers of inflammation can include:

1. Imbalance in our body's acid-base status (pH)
2. The back-up of the inflammation process itself (chemical mediators)
3. Any number of stress chemicals (fight or flight hormones)

When everyday pain, stiffness or discomfort exists, but triggers from a mechanical source are either minimal or nonexistent, sometimes there is what could be considered "concomitant,"[27] coincidental, or simultaneous low-grade inflammatory activity in neighboring organ systems. When part of an organ system, or group of

---

27. The term "concomitant" refers to something that is "naturally accompanying or associated."

tissues related to body systems other than our muscles and joints, experiences inflammatory stress and irritation of its own, it can cause us to become more vulnerable to mechanical forms of strain in those related or neighboring structures. Recall what happens to the neighboring areas next to the treadmill when the treadmill room becomes overwhelmed with inflammation—sometimes the first signal to us that inflammation exists inside the body is when those neighboring structures become uncomfortable enough to complain (Figure 8.1).

One very common example of "complaining" neighboring structures happens in association with a woman's period. From mid-cycle—when the egg is released—to the day she starts her period is a time that is accompanied by a greater tendency for inflammation[li,lii,liii]—body-wide but often more obvious in the areas near the uterus and ovaries. This inflammatory reaction from increased tissue activity that is often related to the second half of the menstrual cycle (roughly, the two weeks before menstrual flow starts) can result in lower back pain. Many women will tell you that this is one way that they know they are about to start the flow part of their period (or in some cases that they are ovulating)—they will start to feel some lower back soreness, aching or stiffness. Based on what we know about inflammation, it's not unreasonable to suppose that this lower back pain is related in some way to the neighboring flare-up—either from the spill-over effect or the mechanical stress of the inflammation-related "traffic jam." Remember, when things swell from the back-up of inflammatory fluids, there will be physical pressure as well as chemical irritation on all surrounding tissues.

Not every woman has the same associated symptoms, and this is a perfect example of the great variation from body to body in our tendency to become inflamed as well as individual tolerance for inflammation. So, think back to the image of the treadmill walkers. Two people doing the same speed of walking or running for the same length of time on the treadmill can show very different signs of stress—depending on fitness level and a whole bunch of other factors that are unique to their chemical, mechanical and emotional make up. But the fact that the treadmill is a source of stress remains indisputable.

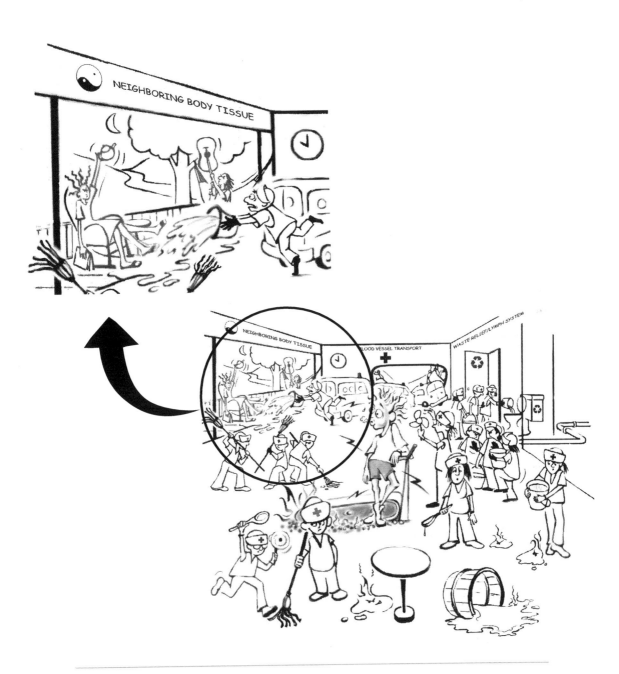

FIGURE 8.1 THE EFFECT OF BUILT-UP WASTE AND INFLAMMATION ON THE NEIGHBORING BODY TISSUES: The result of stressed or injured tissue in the body always has the potential of affecting neighboring structures if the waste and inflammation is allowed to linger even after the cause of stress is removed.

Another interesting lower back pain situation that can arise from something nonmechanical and that is well documented among conventional medical resources is the lower back pain associated with something called prostatitis.[liv] This is usually acute inflammation of the prostate gland in younger men, but certainly the lower back pain that is listed in the medical reference books as a commonly associated symptom is not due to any mechanical accident or injury. It is only seen in conjunction with the inflamed prostate. Again, it's the neighboring tissues (of the lower back) that are taking a bit of a hit for the inflammatory process going on in areas nearby (the prostate in this case).

One more very common example of pain from complaining neighboring structures is related to a concern that patients sometimes have when they come to see me about lower back pain. It's not unusual for me to hear, "Do you think it's my kidneys?" Almost everyone has heard that sometimes kidney problems manifest as back pain. It's true, but luckily I have never seen someone with acute kidney stone–related back pain. This kind of pain is usually so severe that, by the time the back hurts there are often other more severe symptoms that would land you in an urgent care facility first. Again, the mechanism for this intimate relationship between organ system and musculoskeletal system is very likely via the influence of neighboring tissue inflammation. The location of the kidneys just happens to be quite a bit closer to the structures of the back than many other abdominal organs, which might be why this has become a more commonly known association with back pain.

A less well-documented pain syndrome that I do see regularly in my practice is a sudden and severe stiff neck, particularly at the beginning of upper respiratory infection or right before the start of any cold symptoms. I attribute this to the massive sudden onslaught in the lymph tissue and vessels around the head and neck as they start to work on breaking down the invading virus. This extra load chemically and sometimes mechanically (via the pressure from the enlarged lymph nodes) can cause the neighboring neck muscles to become inflamed and stiff—seemingly out of the blue. In my opinion, it's also not out of the question for someone with severe seasonal allergy to experience an increase in neck discomfort as their offending allergen is suddenly blooming and on the rise. It's certainly an association I see often, and the mechanism makes sense.

A healthy body is constantly tackling viruses and allergens before we can catch any wind of it. It's only when our system is *overwhelmed* by the unbalanced load that we exhibit and experience symptoms. So, just because you don't feel under the weather doesn't mean that your lymph nodes and vessels aren't a hub of activity— busily breaking down and eliminating garbage. When that activity gets rowdy, it can exert pressure (mechanical and chemical) on the surrounding structures. What follows are examples of how Ed, Charlene and Billie all experienced some effects from neighboring inflammation.

A situation related to back-up at the lymph nodes:

BILLIE, our 52-year-old office worker who unsuspectingly woke with a stiff neck, is a prime example of this sort of mechanical reaction to inflammation that can be going on just beneath the surface. The most common idea people have about waking with a stiff neck is that they must have just "slept wrong." It's possible that the pillow ended up in a weird place that night or maybe the position for the head and neck wasn't ideal, but often enough, the morning time stiff neck sufferers are waking in a position which they sleep in all the time—so why the pain now? Again, we're looking at that last-drop-in-the-bucket analogy. If you fill it to the brim and then add one more drop —in this case, engorged lymph vessels—to a collection of tense muscles and a stressed immune system, you have yourself a perfect recipe for a frozen neck. It's an over-reaction for sure but not uncommon.

Because stiffness = inflammation, Billie doesn't get to leave my office without some ice applied to the neck and a stern warning: Under no circumstances should she give in to the urge to stretch the neck! Going back to the types of stressors that cause inflammation, you'll recall that lengthening is one of the chief stressors. When the neck is already dealing with inflammation, the last thing you want to do is add another stressor by moving your head farther away from center—unless you want to see the neck muscles spasm even more. (See Chapter 2 on mechanical triggers.)

Is there yet more fallout from PMS?

CHARLENE, our dancer-yoga instructor, also occasionally ended up in my office—even before giving birth to her son—for neck pain that spanned from her shoulder blade up to her head. It never failed that, when this issue flared up, it happened during the one to two weeks between ovulation and her period. She would not be doing anything new in her dance or yoga practice, and yet invariably, this area of her body, that for her is structurally vulnerable, would flare up while she was doing things that she had diligently trained her body to do and had done hundreds of times before without strain.

The reasons for Charlene's pre-existing vulnerability in this area have to do with a previous injury, complicated by structural asymmetry that is unique to how her body developed—in combination with how she expresses herself through movement and everyday posture. We all have these vulnerable areas. None of us is perfectly symmetrical and, even despite our best efforts, we can end up with one group of muscles that are weaker than others. None of this is a problem until, again, that last drop in the inflammation bucket. For Charlene, before pregnancy, this neck pain flare-up occurred regularly during the last half of her menstrual cycle, which is classically when I tend to see "mysterious" injuries like this in my female patients. There is some evidence that due to certain hormone level changes at this time, there is more "systemic," or, in other words, body-wide, inflammation.[iv] An increase in body-wide inflammation can be all it takes to tip the scales and throw off the balance of what seemed to be working without pain until that point.

Could your coffee be injuring you?

ED is the patient who coincidentally noted a possible association between the timing of a spike in his coffee intake and the back strain/sprain that he came to see me for. When I discussed this connection in Chapter 3, I was asking you to consider the postural changes that a painful belly[28] would cause, thereby contributing to the mechanical stress. It's typical for low-grade abdominal discomfort to cause collapse in the torso from even just slightly doubling over—as would be natural for most of us with belly pain.

The coffee connection also presented the possibility of pH-related pain due to its acidifying effect, but the other aspect of abdominal discomfort when considering chemical causes of nearby pain—whether it's because of coffee or constipation or irritable bowel issues—is the chemical effect of that inflammation-related visceral (related to the internal organs) pain on the neighboring structures. I often see combinations of presenting symptoms like this, for example:

1. Acid reflux with left upper back and shoulder blade pain (the area right behind the stomach and esophagus)
2. Constipation and left-sided lower back pain[29] (the area behind the last part of the colon)
3. Gallbladder attacks preceded by right-sided upper back and shoulder blade pain (the area right behind the gallbladder and liver)

---

28. Ed was experiencing stomach pain after drinking coffee.

29. More often than not, constipation alone causes subtle postural changes and mechanical stress local to the lower back rather than inflammation.

These combinations aren't always obvious because the visceral inflammation and dysfunction are often low grade and largely asymptomatic (no noticeable symptoms), except for the associated or referred pain that sometimes gets mistaken for back pain. When I delve further into someone's health history, I often find those subtle connections.

So, to keep everyday pain at bay, we should all be working at bringing our insides in synch with our outsides as well as vice versa. This means it is important to find *physical/mechanical* balance in how we move against gravity through our everyday life. In addition, we should also consider finding *chemical* balance to help decrease the chances of developing inflammation, whether that be a raging flare-up or a low-grade, simmering situation. As we've seen, imbalance in one area (chemical, mechanical or emotional) can be associated with increased vulnerability to strain in one of the other categories. The question is: How do we find that body chemistry balance?

In order to foster a greater tolerance for those inflammatory chemical fluctuations that are difficult to control, like that of the menstrual cycle or the seasonality of environmental allergens, we need to learn how to manipulate the chemical triggers that *are* within our control. The best we can do is to avoid as many of these controllable triggers as possible. In other words, to exert control over chemical triggers that we cannot avoid, the answer is often to simply lighten our load as much as possible of *other* chemical irritants that we *can* avoid. Remember, it's the slow cumulative effect of millions of tiny drops in the bucket that brings it to the brim. The ways we know of that can decrease the chemical stress of body-wide inflammation naturally are[lvi]:

- Taking in enzymes, herbs and anti-inflammatory foods
- Engaging in anything that facilitates waste elimination, like body movement, drinking water, eating fiber, and producing sweat (preferably by exercise and not fear or negative stress)

What this boils down to is taking control of the balance between "garbage in" and "garbage out".

We can start finding inner chemical balance by addressing all of those invisible offenders in our food and air ("garbage in"). Once again, let's revisit those three main chemical triggers of inflammation:

1. pH (our biologic acidity levels)
2. Molecules produced by injured tissue (chemical mediators of inflammation)
3. Chemistry of emotional stress (stress addiction)

All three of these things have the potential to push our physiology out of balance. We can influence them by addressing our internal and external environment. The air we breathe and the things we ingest, both liquid and solid, are the sources of potential tissue stress that may challenge our acid-base balance and/or add to our allergen load, which can stress the immune system. When our immune system is managing molecules that aren't completely compatible with our chemistry, it undergoes stress (Diagram 8.1). The process our immune system goes through to protect us from viruses, bad bacteria or allergens involves an influx of activity into our lymph system (part of the body's sewer network) as the sewage-treatment plants go into high gear due to the additional load of "foreign invaders" that need to be broken down for elimination. Remember, when there is a back-up in any one of our elimination systems, inflammation can result. Inflammation that is allowed to build up and overwhelm us will result in pain. A low level of simmering inflammation will set us up to be more vulnerable and to react more easily to other body stressors.

You may require professional assistance to determine what causes chemical stress for *your* body. With the help of a health care provider who can order the right tests or guide you through the process of elimination, you can find out both:

1. Which allergens *your* body has the most difficulty with—airborne or food-related (pain due to excess waste accumulation and tissue stress)
2. Which foods might be creating an acidic environment (pain due to pH imbalance)

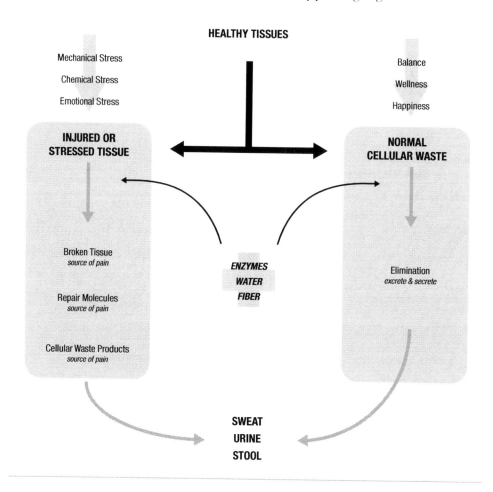

DIAGRAM 8.1 COMPLEXITIES OF WASTE ELIMINATION: Natural elimination of waste from our cells and tissues is sometimes complicated by additional work dealing with damaged tissue fragments, used-up repair molecules and waste products of the repair process.

These two categories of influences on your chemistry can be what are causing you to harbor a constant low level of inflammation. There are some commonly known allergens and acid-forming foods that I would encourage you to learn more about. Please refer to the Appendix for further reading on these subjects, but these topics will also be revisited in Volume Two, which will be dedicated to outlining specific strategies for buffering your body against mechanical, chemical and emotional stressors.

If you want to become "fire proof" by managing your chemistry, here are some ideas for how to address the three main chemical triggers of inflammation and pain.

Recall from Chapter 3 that pain can arise from a migration toward acidity in the body tissues. Things that can cause this sort of shift toward a more acidic pH are:

- Natural build-up of **cellular waste**
- **Tissue-repair response** in an area of injured or stressed tissue
- **Damaged tissue** itself from stress or injury

There are three main factors that can either contribute to the build-up of excess cellular waste (from both healthy tissue and stressed tissue) or can result in the accumulation of troublemaking molecular byproducts (from stressed body tissue-repair response and presence of damaged tissue particles). These are factors that we *can* exert some control over:

- Food
- Breath
- Allergens: food and environment

How can we exert control over these three factors?

1. Arm yourself with **enzymes**—through nutrients and food
2. Fix your essential fatty acid ratio (omega 6 to **omega 3**[lvii])—through food and fish oil
3. **Detoxify and eliminate**—making the most of targeted nutrients via motion and breath to drive the efficient production of sweat, urine and stool

Take and Make Your Enzymes!

These little golden nuggets of cellular warfare do the dirty work needed to diffuse many waste products of everyday tissue metabolism as well as by-products of stressed and inflamed tissue. We make our own army of enzymes thanks to the pancreas and gallbladder, but sometimes when the body is under attack by waste and toxins, our natural enzyme production capacity is just not enough to keep up. When this is the case, we can take in extra enzymes through supplements or food. There are three categories of enzymes that we need in order to break down the three basic groups of waste products: amylase to break down carbohydrates, proteases to break down proteins and fatty wastes and lipases to break down fats or lipids.

If you prefer to eat whole food instead of taking supplements, you'll find amylase in sprouts like alfalfa. Proteases can be found in papaya and pineapple. Food sources of lipase include lentils, oats and avocado.[lviii] To support the body's own abilities to produce and release all three of these digestive enzymes, it's been found that eating bitter herbs is extremely effective.[lix]

Balance Your Essential Fatty Acids!

It's actually these behind-the-scenes essential fatty acids in our food and their balance in the body that determines how inflamed we might become or how well we may handle inflammation[lx] when it comes our way. They are called "essential" because, unlike the enzymes, our body does not manufacture these on its own. We need to eat them in our diet. These essential fatty acids fall into two main groups: omega 3 and omega 6 fats. We need both in order to drive many metabolic reactions in the body that benefit our handling of neuron signaling and coordination of the inflammation pathways. Our body does this by disassembling the fatty acids that we eat into these two very special components: eicosapentaenoic acid (EPA) and docosahexaenioc acid (DHA).

EPA and DHA are the real heroes in this story. They help us make something called "resolvins," which decrease inflammation. They also form an important part of the cell membrane that facilitates nerve signaling—improving communication among body tissues and your brain. In addition, they help to control the level of triglycerides (low density lipoprotein), which are associated with increased inflammation.[lxi] Raising omega 3 levels (decreasing the omega 6:3 ratio[lxii]) is what leads to more available EPA and DHA. We *can* make EPA and DHA from omega 6 oils, but it's much harder work for the body and with significantly less yield than just eating more omega 3.

Sources of omega 6 include grains, seeds, nuts and many other plant sources that in our modern diet, occur often in overabundance. Sources of the coveted *omega 3* include fish oil, fish oil and more fish oil. Fish is the only source of omega 3 fat that we don't have to make by laboriously converting omega 6.

The optimal ratio[lxiii] of omega 6 to omega 3 is much lower when considering best-case scenario inflammation control. For example, the omega 6:3 ratio of 4:1 has been shown to effectively decrease risk of heart disease (heart disease has, of course, been strongly linked to inflammation). Inflammatory conditions like rheumatoid arthritis respond better to a ratio between 2 and 3:1. Early humans were found to show a 1:1 ratio of omega 6 to omega 3 intake. Unfortunately, today our intake is between a 15:1 and 16:1 ratio of omega 6 to omega 3. This modern-day dominance of omega 6 is extremely inflammatory but is a natural result of a diet high in grains (in other words, carbohydrates), seeds (vegetable oils) and nuts in the absence of adequate leafy greens, berries and fish. This is the real reason why so many of us benefit from lowering our carbohydrate intake. It's not just about gluten intolerance. Avoiding carbohydrates is a smart move but not enough to change the omega 6:3 ratio. Leafy greens need to increase by leaps and bounds and fish oil needs to be considered.[30] There is much controversy around the intake and commercialization of fish sources due to rising concentrations of heavy-metal toxicity contamination of our environment.[lxiv] Find some suggestions for further reading in the Appendix.

Detoxify and Eliminate!

The word "detox" has become very trendy and many of us have come to associate the term with any variety of radical juice-fasting types of diet methods. The truth is that our body is actually naturally detoxifying us every day all day long. When you move your body you are effectively powering the hydraulic pumping of fluids from your tissues and organs to the kidneys, skin and colon, shuttling garbage toward the exits. Breathing is a significant driver of this process both via the movement it creates and

---

30. Many fish are contaminated with heavy metals. It's important to eat wild fish and fish on the list of least contaminated (for further reading, see the Appendix). If taking fish oil supplements, you should look for those that are "molecularly distilled" to help ensure toxin-free purity.

the gas exchange that happens. Carbon dioxide is acidic, and expelling it in exchange for oxygen is chemically detoxifying. This means when you breathe, sweat, urinate and have a bowel movement, you are in effect carrying out an essential step in the natural detoxification process! Your liver and kidneys and skin are primary detoxifying organs. They filter, disassemble or do their best to at least disable invaders that don't belong.

What *you* can do to help the process above and beyond simply breathing, sweating, peeing and pooping is to:

1. **Avoid** exposing yourself to new toxins
2. **Move** to mechanically get the garbage out
3. **Flush** it out with fluids and fiber

Avoid!

Decreasing the work load on your organs makes their job easier and makes them more efficient at what they do best. What you can do to help decrease the load on these organs of elimination is to watch your intake of *new* irritants, toxins, allergens , among others, via air and food. Give your body a chance to deal with the toxins and allergens already on board. A brief overview of what this might include would be chemicals, fumes, any artificial ingredients—either flavor or color or fragrance—and preservatives. A general rule for identifying things that the body considers toxic would be if the ingredients of something going on your skin, in your mouth or through your airways isn't listed in everyday words that you're familiar with. If all you see on a label is names of chemical compounds, then it's probably going to tax your systems of elimination.

Move!

Movement powers the mechanical pumping of fluids carrying waste through your body to places where it can be dumped and eliminated. Exercise will cause an increase in breath rate that will get the stale stagnant air out of the bottom of your lungs and replace it with oxygen rich air. Oxygen feeds your body tissues. When you're in too much pain to exercise safely, another way to power this pumping mechanism for detoxification is to receive bodywork of some kind. Trained hands can help not only loosen up tight muscles, which *feels* good, but they also help move the garbage in your body to help get it out. This is why sometimes we get sore after being worked on in a similar way to after we exercise.

Flush!

If your body is dehydrated, moving molecules of waste becomes more difficult. You can exercise and get bodywork, but you'll be much less effective at pushing the garbage out if your fluids are the consistency of mud instead of water. Water will improve how well garbage moves out of the muscles and spaces in between, but fiber is what escorts many "unsavory characters" or "undesirable" molecules out through the digestive tract. We all know we need to eat fiber to be able to have good bowel movements but it's more than that. Fiber literally binds to the garbage in our gut and drags it out as it passes through. It truly cleans up. How you take fiber—by food or supplementing—is tricky and very individual. I would recommend consulting with a naturopathic doctor before you radically change your fiber intake. Some people will get stopped up and others may experience excessive loosening of the stool initially, and both of these results can potentially cause more inflammation.

Possible Chemical Sources of Pain and Inflammation By Location

What follows now is a section divided into upper and lower body regions. If you have pain in the upper half of your body, you can find under the heading of "Upper Body" all of the possible organ systems that may be subtly involved with your pain, based on

"A low level of simmering inflammation will set us up to be more vulnerable and to react more easily to other body stressors."

the idea that inflammation in one area can cause neighboring tissues to experience pain and vice versa (Diagrams 8.2 and 8.3). The same applies if you happen to be looking at "Lower Body"-related structures (Diagrams 8.4 and 8.5). This is information you can use to serve as your starting point as you begin finding out how to keep your pain from happening again *if* part of it is happening because of a body chemistry imbalance or vulnerability. You'll also see a diagram of visceral (related to the internal organs) pain referral patterns, which are another means by which pain can link an organ to a muscle. Many structures share common nerve fibers and branches, so, when one of these areas is in distress, the other ones fed by the same family of nerves can experience discomfort as well.

If your pain is in the upper half of your body, here are *some* of the neighboring structures and systems that might be out of balance:

Upper body :

- ✓ Neck
- ✓ Shoulder
- ✓ Shoulder blade
- ✓ Mid-back
- ✓ Torso
- ✓ Ribs

Remember, this is just a suggestion to consider the *possibility* that the structures near the area of pain may also be under stress. Decreasing the stress in your neighboring tissues can in some cases help the injured area to recover more quickly. Ideas for how to care for different organ systems under stress can come from any number of alternative health providers, like naturopaths, chiropractors, acupuncturists, herbalists and nutritionists. These different therapeutic avenues and some highlights about some helpful herbs and nutrients will be addressed in the second chapter of Volume Two in looking at chemical repair. The Appendix will also provide further reading.

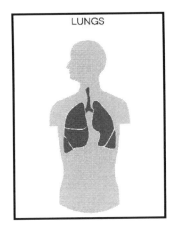
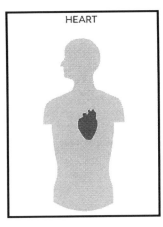
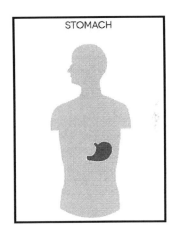
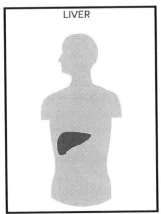
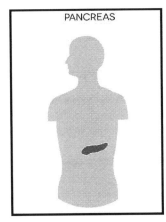

DIAGRAM 8.2 UPPER BODY–RELATED ORGAN SYSTEMS: Shown here are nearby organ systems to consider when you have upper body pain.

Examples of Imbalance That Might Accompany and Add to Pain in the Upper Body

- Sinus congestion/allergy
- Head cold
- Heartburn/gastric reflux
- Asthma
- Cough

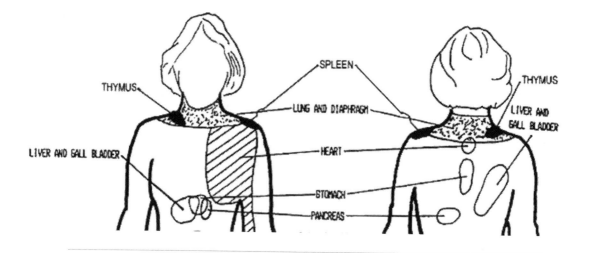

DIAGRAM 8.3 UPPER BODY VISCERAL REFERRAL PATTERNS

If your pain is in the lower half of your body, here are *some* of the neighboring structures and systems that might be out of balance:

Lower body :
- ✓ Mid-back
- ✓ Torso
- ✓ Ribs
- ✓ Lower back
- ✓ Hip
- ✓ Buttocks

Remember, this is just a suggestion to consider the *possibility* that the structures near the area of pain may also be under stress. Decreasing the stress in your neighboring tissues can in some cases help the injured area to recover more quickly. Ideas for how to care for different organ systems under stress can come from any number of alternative health providers like naturopaths, chiropractors, acupuncturists, herbalists and nutritionists. These different therapeutic avenues and some highlights about some helpful herbs and nutrients will be addressed in the second chapter in Volume Two in looking at chemical repair. The Appendix will also provide further reading.

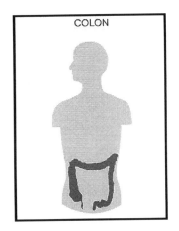
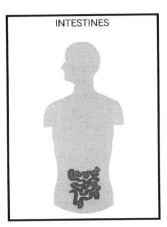
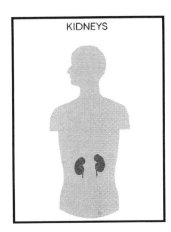
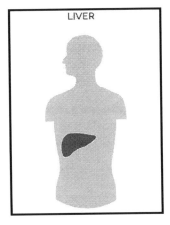
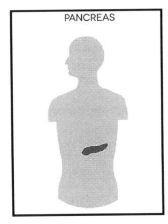

DIAGRAM 8.4 LOWER BODY-RELATED ORGAN SYSTEMS: Shown here are nearby organ systems to consider when you have upper body pain.

Examples of Imbalance That Might Accompany and Add to Pain in the Lower Body

- Intestinal back-up/constipation
- Intestinal inflammation/gas build-up, bloating
- Ovulation, build-up to period
- Gynecological fibroids/cysts
- Urinary tract inflammation
- Prostatitis

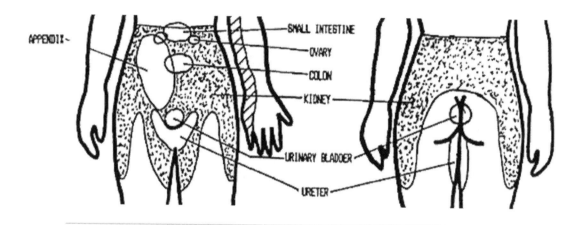

DIAGRAM 8.5 LOWER BODY VISCERAL REFERRAL PATTERNS

When you decide you've found a relationship between your pain and your related body organs or systems of the nearby regions, what do you do about it? If you've already explored and implemented the natural detoxification tactics to help your body decrease its inflammatory load but you're still feeling pain, you might need a little extra help.

Hands-on bodywork techniques like massage, chiropractic and Chinese medicine are not only for feeling better; they can make your body function better by optimizing molecular communication between cells. There are a lot of bodywork methods that, while addressing muscles and joints from the outside, will also profoundly affect the function of the organ systems nearby, not only because blood flow and

"To exert control over chemical triggers that we cannot avoid, the answer is often to simply lighten our load as much as possible of other chemical irritants that we can avoid."

drainage is being positively affected, but via networks of relay points that may work entirely on an electromagnetic or neurochemical level. For example, there are neurolymphatic points in and among our superficial structure—the top surface layers covering the body and contained by the skin and fascia. These points (originally named Chapman reflexes)[lxv] were found to act via a viscera-somatic[31] reflex mechanism, which affects the influence that our sympathetic nervous system (our control panel of the fight or flight reaction) has on related organ systems (see the Appendix for further reading).

Another very well mapped-out access system (another kind of control panel or motherboard) to our body energy and function is known as the *meridian system* in acupuncture and Chinese medicine. Meridians and neurolymphatic points may very well be related.[lxvi] We'll revisit these modalities and more in the next two volumes of this book series, as I help you explore the repair, rebuilding and prevention of damage from the inflammation of everyday pain.

On the other hand, you may also help optimize your organ system functions by paying attention to your body's chemical inflammatory stressors. Sometimes just making sure to avoid new exposure to possible inflammation triggers is enough to allow the body to clean itself out and allow all organ systems to function with greater ease. When left to its own devices and fed clean fuel, the body can be a very effective self-healing machine. Think of what happens with scrapes and cuts on our skin.

---

31. Having to do with the "viscera" (known as the organ systems) and the "soma" (the body structure).

These things fix themselves in no time and with no help from us—as long as we don't continually pick at the scab. Repeatedly exposing ourselves to mechanical, chemical or emotional irritants is the equivalent of picking at a scab—not allowing it to heal.

An important thing to remember when you become tempted to think about your body in compartments: the reality is that all compartments are related in some way. Everything bears a common thread or two, and sometimes that's literally by the shared walls of structures that happen to be in direct contact with each other. The common link could also be via shared blood supply, nerve pathways or even common embryologic tissue from how we developed in utero.

Our nervous system (neuroendocrine system, to be more accurate) is the great unifier and coordinates much of how the body functions and responds. This means that, no matter how isolated you think your pain is, it's possible that your brain (neuro) and your hormones (endocrine) are making it a body-wide issue as they engage in their complex call-and-response dance between all tissues and cells of the body. It could be that there's a larger issue of imbalance that your pain is trying to signal you about. The term "hormones" refers to more than just the commonly associated hormones of sex and reproduction. Hormones are signaling and communication molecules can be found everywhere in our body and come customized for each tissue and organ system. These molecules are busy coordinating everything from digestion to sleep by a complex network of neuroendocrine signaling. This means the condition of your nervous system can play a big role in how well your organ functioning is being coordinated.

At any given moment we can find ourselves at one end of the scale or another between sympathetic (high alert) and parasympathetic (relaxed) states. Too often, modern life lends itself to keeping us stuck in a state of sustained sympathetic tone. This means we get stuck in the indecision of the fight-or-flight response with nowhere to go. Our sympathetic nervous system response is a fantastic survival tool and designed for short spurts—"phasic" activity. Unfortunately, when we get stuck in a sustained version of heightened alert (or "tonic" sympathetic activity) we become worn down and less able to deal with any and all stressors—mechanical, chemical and emotional.

The way we experience the state of "sustained sympathetic tone" is physical. The way we get to that point is emotional.

CHAPTER 9

Fire Proof Emotions and Mindset

THE BEST WAY TO TAKE CONTROL of our sympathetic/parasympathetic states is to pay attention to our emotional balance.

Let's go back for a moment to that joke about: "Well, if it hurts to do _____, then stop doing it!" In considering the ironic wisdom behind that silly-sounding advice, what I find striking is the sometimes vigorous resistance I encounter when gently broaching with patients that very idea. If it hurts to do something, we really *do* just have to stop it. But apparently it's not so easy for many of us to accept that there are some basic things that we have to modify about our daily life to accommodate periods of pain and dysfunction. The association with being perceived as "defective" or "disabled" in some way is for many of us a hard pill to swallow, but are these sorts of adjectives actually applicable when dealing with everyday pain? Not at all, yet at some level we can't help but struggle with reconciling our worth and our physical abilities, which makes this common, anxious association reaction perfectly understandable.

How does pain and physical hindrance make *you* feel? Some of us experience fear. Some get angry. Some stew about it. All of these different emotions can profoundly affect your recovery and the rest of your health.

In Eastern medicine, within the vast realm of ancient Eastern philosophies, there are old ideas and principles that have been developed over the centuries that connect certain body regions and organ systems with specific emotions. Could it be that emotions out of balance lead to organ system dysfunction or vice versa? Or perhaps the emotional imbalance simply coexists with the physiologic imbalance? The fact is that a relationship between the two is acknowledged as a given in many parts of the world. Eastern perspectives in health have always recognized the emotions as an integral part of overall health, whether through the system of chakras—energy centers of the body—or the meridian system of energy points and channels. Based on the crudest of interpretations of a few Chinese medicine principles, we can roughly summarize rudimentary connections between these five primary emotions and how they relate to anatomy as follows[lxvii]:

lung   ↔   sorrow
liver   ↔   anger
heart   ↔   joy
spleen   ↔   worry
kidney   ↔   fear

(It should be noted that organ names in this list are used to refer to a wider system of body meridians, which ultimately do affect the organ in question but in a subtle way—not necessarily in the linear, mainstream medical sense where full blown pathology would be evident.[32])

As with all other stressors, it's the overall imbalance of these emotions that can be associated with stress at any particular part of the meridian system. Emotions are seen as occurring on one of these five areas as listed above—each along an infinite spectrum. For example, an *excess* of "joy" would be what we might consider mania in the extreme, and this can be just as damaging to the heart meridian or heart energy as can be a *depletion* of joy, which we might see as depression in the other extreme.

---

32. Meridians are defined in acupuncture and Chinese medicine as a series of pathways in the body along which vital energy flows. There are twelve such pathways associated with specific organs.

This simplistic statement does no justice to the complexity of how the five elements and organ systems interrelate. One is never affected without consequences to all five other systems in some way (Diagram 9.1).

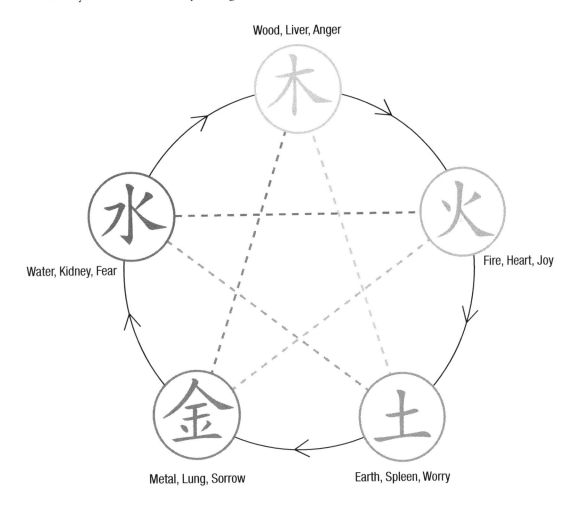

DIAGRAM 9.1 EMOTIONS IN CHINESE MEDICINE: The lines and arrows depicted here show the inter-relatedness between the five organ systems and their corresponding emotions assigned by Eastern medicine theory. The direction of each arrow shows the direction of influence by the imbalance of any one organ system, element or emotion. Excess of any one can contribute to both an excess (overactivity), or depletion (underactivity) of numerous other organ systems and corresponding emotions. The art of Chinese medicine relies heavily upon the under-standing of the intricacies of this inter-relatedness.

What's significant here is that most Eastern styles of medicine pay just as much attention to the patient's state of mind as to the state of his or her tissues and organs. This insight and acknowledgment of the whole person rather than reducing us to our individual body parts is based on healing methods centuries old that survive because they work.

There do exist more modern Western interpretations of the connection between pain and state of mind, such as that promoted by Louise Hay (known for her support of and pioneering work with mind-body centered resource centers in the United States). These correlations most likely have their roots in ancient Eastern thought connecting a wide spectrum of the five basic emotions and elements with body regions and tissue systems. While there is a growing body of research in the field of "psychoneuroimmunology,"[33] I urge you to review this information with an open mind and cautious perspective. There is danger in thinking too rigidly that we have an exclusive, internal locus of control.[34] We must do the best we can to control what we can—and there is indeed much that *is* within our control—but there are also things in life that are best let go of. The trick is knowing where that line is. You can't go wrong if you make sure to always be kind to yourself. Be accepting of circumstances outside of your control. See the hopefulness in the information presented here but beware any crushing sense of responsibility to take it *all* upon yourself. What *is* up to you and only you is finding a peaceful perspective and acceptance. It's our tendency to struggle against what *is* that causes emotional imbalance.

The mind-body connection is indisputable. Circumstances are sometimes out of our control, but how we face these circumstances shapes our experience, and that is something completely within our control (Figures 9.1 and 9.2). Again, you'll find in the Appendix references for further reading by other authorities on the subject, like Joan Borysenko, PhD, who has advanced degrees in medical science and psychology, as well as Bruce Lipton, PhD, a stem cell biologist and author of *Biology of Belief*. There will also be further exploration of this mind-body connection with pain and inflammation in Chapter 6 of *Volume Two: Fix the Fire Damage.*

---

33. *Merriam-Webster's* dictionary notes that the term didn't come into use until 1982, so that tells you how young the field really is!

34. Locus of control refers to the extent to which individuals believe that they can control events affecting them. Understanding of the concept was developed by Julian B. Rotter in 1954, and it has since become an aspect of personality studies.

Rough Summary of Some Ideas to Consider About Pain From the Mind-Body Perspective

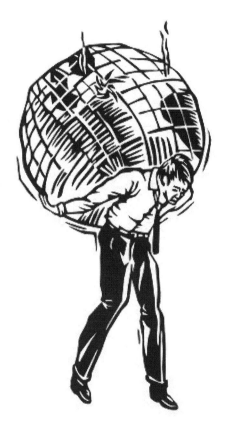

UPPER BODY

Having pain in your upper body?

Are your arms shoulders and neck bearing the "weight of the world"? Are you "shouldering" too much responsibility?

LOWER BODY

Having pain in your lower back, legs or feet?

Are there big changes in your life that you are either working hard toward or meeting resistance about? Finding it difficult to move forward?

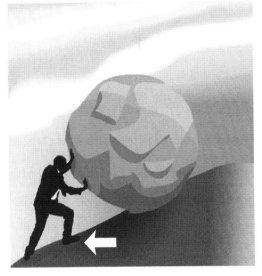

FIGURE 9.1 THE WEIGHT OF THE WORLD: Upper body (top).
FIGURE 9.2 MOVING FORWARD: Lower body (bottom).

When you make efforts to buffer yourself emotionally (as well as chemically and mechanically), you ensure your very best chance at becoming ultimately "fire proof"—resistant to the fire of inflammation. Developing an emotional buffer in addition to the mechanical and chemical buffers will be your very best bet at keeping everyday pain at bay.

> "You can't go wrong if you make sure to always be kind to yourself."

Now would be a good time to ask: "How do you use this information about emotions to keep the everyday pain from happening again?" It will have to involve addressing three aspects of emotion:

1. Stress
2. Self-image
3. Worldview

Stress

To address stress, we should be aware that the kind of emotional stress that leads to inflammation starts in the "reptilian brain"[35] and has an extremely reasonable survival purpose. We can't just tell ourselves to stop being stressed when it's based on a legitimate biologic need. What we have to do is find a way to provide an outlet, an opportunity for our physical body to release the chemical storm of this very sensible but misplaced fear response. When we find ways to release and redirect this kind of stress, we will effectively be stepping out of the way to allow our body's natural processes to take place.

It's not often socially acceptable to scream and cry when we feel biologically stressed like we can do as infants, and in fact it's probably not helpful chemically

---

35. The term "reptilian brain" refers to our most primitive brain functions. For an entertaining and educational discussion on the topic, read Verstynen and Voytek's *Do Zombies Dream of Undead Sheep?: A Neuroscientific View of the Zombie Brain*, published in 2014.

"It's our tendency to struggle against what is that causes emotional imbalance."

to do it for prolonged periods of time. Have you ever noticed that when you scratch an itchy insect bite, it tends to just get itchier? In the medical world this is referred to—in not-so-sophisticated terms—as the "itch scratch cycle."[lxviii] A similar thing can happen with the fear and anger behind stress. The more time we spend screaming and crying—whether that's literally or figuratively—the more we effectively scratch that stress-itch and reinforce it. Okay, so the answer we've come up with as adults is to bottle up—scream and cry on the *inside* instead of letting it out. But there *are* other ways to cope.

Of course, this begs the question: "How, then?" How do we allow the natural processing of this fear response? Here are some ideas:

1. Exercise!
2. Sleep!
3. Shift...your outlook on life!

Exercise!

This doesn't have to be of the butt-kicking variety in order to achieve positive effects on stress. In fact, you should be careful how much stress your exercise habits *themselves* might be causing. Sometimes vigorous sustained exercise just encourages the production and release of destructive stress hormones.[lxix] Your mindset during exercise is also important. Are you enjoying the activity? Are you focusing on how terrible you feel, or on how much you'd rather be doing something else? Then maybe exercise is not the best way for you to decompress. Exercise is important for many physiologic reasons, but it can also be possible to find perspective and gain control over stress by simply connecting with nature. Hiking in the woods, for example, can provide a form of moving meditation that triggers anti-depressant effects from the side-to-side eye motion required during that kind of walking.[lxx] "Quiet time" is something you can experience while moving about gently in nature, or you can experience it in the gym getting a sweat going, with your headphones on. Anything that provides focus and reflection inward is something you can use to recalibrate the mind.

Recalibration of the mind and emotions is ultimately the result of a chemical shift in your brain and body. The tool that leads you to that shift can be something like aerobic activity, which studies have shown does indeed change brain chemicals.[lxxi] The shift can also come from any experience that elicits a phenomenon called "flow." Mihaly Czikszentmihalyi is considered a top researcher on the topic of "positive psychology,"[lxxii] and he's the one who came up with the concept of "flow."[lxxiii] Whether it's through work, the physical effort of exercise or by sitting still on a park bench listening to birds, "flow" is the experience of effortless concentration and joy that comes from complete immersion into an experience. When we find flow, time becomes irrelevant. When you find flow in your life, you will have found an appropriate redirect for your stress, a way to control and decrease it.

Sleep!

This phenomenon is still a bit of a scientific mystery to researchers, but there is increasing evidence that the amount and quality of sleep correlates with stress levels.[lxxiv] It has been found to be important in warding off stress,[lxxv] which surely is no surprise to you. Not only does sleep make us kinder and gentler people, but based on the connection between stress and inflammation, it's safe to say that sleep may very well be linked to inflammatory levels in the body.[lxxvi]

The problem with sleep is that it is completely undervalued in many modern cultures.[lxxvii] During college, it's not uncommon to boast and be rewarded for the fewest hours of sleep or missing entire nights of sleep. Another example of pandemic proportions: Glorifying sleep deprivation is what seems to still be a prestigious rite of passage for medical residents as these young doctors begin their hospital careers. With this sort of social undercurrent, the rest of us learn to lose respect for the ritual and allow ourselves to fall out of practice with this regenerative six to nine hours a night.

It's very important to consciously restore the routine around sleep and even consider making daytime napping a regular habit. Twenty minutes of rest with eyes closed may not bring you the deepest brainwaves of nighttime sleep, but has been shown to be close to an optimal rest time needed to recharge the mind.[lxxviii]

Shift!

Shifting your outlook on life is very likely the *least* easy thing to change (and you might not be successful at it until you're getting enough sleep). So many of life's formative experiences happen during early childhood—before we have much say or awareness of these influences, yet they determine how we cope with everyday stress. How you view yourself and your world determines your experience and perception of stressful situations. Your outlook has a lot to do with how you see yourself (your self-image) and how you see others around you in relationship to yourself (your worldview). These things sometimes require us to seek outside help, just like when we are troubleshooting mechanical and chemical aspects of our everyday pain. Outside therapeutic help in the area of emotional balance is sometimes the best way to achieve effective and lasting recalibration of some unhelpful perspectives learned years ago that might have us behaving and reacting on "unconscious autopilot" in unproductive ways. Luckily, the negative stigma attached to psychotherapy is lessening (but not yet gone[lxxix]), becoming more supportive, and access to competent psychologists is becoming easier as the attitudes toward the discipline of mental health change.[lxxx] If you are truly pursuing whole health, having a psychologist on your health care team is just as essential as having a chiropractor, physical therapist, naturopath or an integrative medical doctor.

Self-Image: "I Can Do It" vs. "I'm No Good at This"

How you see yourself and your abilities can change your entire experience of everyday episodes of pain. If your experience of yourself is that you can tackle life obstacles and come out on top, you probably see yourself as capable and self-assured. Someone who feels capable and self-assured is less likely to fall victim to the fear of helplessness that can come from unexpected or unfamiliar sudden pain. On the other hand, if you've only ever seen yourself as unsure and perhaps your self-esteem is not strong, then it's even more important for you to adhere to the recommendations in Section II for pain mitigating measures. You may be more vulnerable to becoming overwhelmed by fear—stressed by the worry that your pain might devolve into a worst case scenario of unknown proportions.

Working on your attitude and outlook about the changes you find yourself having to make in your daily life to accommodate the pain may be easier to accept if you show yourself that you really *can* make changes in your everyday pain—no matter how subtle. The fear of helplessness can sometimes overtake us and paralyze our efforts, but with the tiny windows of empowerment over your pain that can come from taking baby steps that do have a positive effect (like those described in Chapter 5, starting with the stop, drop and roll technique), you become able to recall that you are not actually helpless in this situation. That is a key piece to hold on to during difficult times. You really *can* do it!

Worldview: "Success Is Possible." vs. "Things Will Get Worse No Matter What I Do."

"Worldview" is about how we see the world in relation to us; in other words, what do we see is our place in this world. Our assessment of others gives us context or understanding of ourselves just as much as our understanding of self informs our opinion of others and the world around us. This assessment isn't necessarily accurate, but our perception shapes our reality. Not only does worldview along with self-image become embodied in a postural display (as we discussed briefly in Chapter 4, Figure 4.1), but where our worldview falls on the spectrum of determinism vs. free will influences the outcome of our interactions with others.

Determinism implies that all events, including human action, are ultimately determined by causes outside of our wishes or intentions. This worldview might lead to that sense of helplessness toward pain. It might also lead to a sense of acceptance that results in less stress. Less stress is good, but be careful that your acceptance of everyday pain doesn't turn into complacency, which will most certainly lead to more pain eventually.

If you fall closer to the free-will end of this worldview spectrum, in my opinion you'll be more likely to take control of your everyday pain situation and successfully nip it in the bud. Which end of the spectrum fits you? Which type of person would you rather be? Remember that it's part of a process. Nothing is static. Take time to look at where you are and where you want to go and remember, as long as you're living and breathing, change is not only possible, it's inevitable, so you might as well shape it to suit you! It can be hard work but success *is* possible.

All efforts to improve your health need to come from a place of joy and hope and not as a way to punish yourself or because you feel you "have to"—whether you're working on achieving mechanical, chemical or emotional balance. Remember you're doing it in the quest for optimum functioning—finding that "sweet spot" where you have just enough protective habits in place to help you survive less-than-perfect situations without experiencing pain. The idea is that you don't have to live a perfect life to be pain free, so there's no real reason to get down on yourself for all the imperfections. Instead of looking at yourself as something broken or defective that needs "fixing," remember that life is truly an ongoing adventure! We are all on a continuum with individual strengths and weaknesses that tug and pull at us daily. Everybody, complete with their physical imperfections, is in the same boat, and we're all busy seeking, learning and trying.

Whatever motivates you to be kind to yourself will be your way toward a good outcome. Generally, for long-term, positive results, it's better to be moderate in your goal setting and to pace yourself as you would for a marathon rather than creating unrealistic expectations of how to be "perfect" from this day forward. The quest for "perfection" is a sure way to fail. Perfection is largely an illusion.

We all have ups and downs with our commitments to routine and self-care and the best we can do is to always find a way to try again—start over and keep trying—all with loving forgiveness.

> "When you find flow in your life, you will have found an appropriate re-direct for your stress, a way to control and decrease it."

A Word About Headaches

For some people, head pain can serve as a weathervane of sorts related to the level of acceptable inflammatory stress in the body. In many cases headaches signal imbalance in one or more of the body systems. However, you'll notice a glaring omission in this book about anything directly related to headaches. Head pain *can* be related to neck pain in the relatively straightforward way described in this guide. You might even find that if you apply the information about general everyday pain from this book you might notice a decrease in some types of head pain. However, headaches comprise a much more complex topic that would not be done justice in the context I am asking readers to consider, and it deserves its own book. Many of the principles regarding inflammation and imbalance touched on in *Every Body's Guide to Everyday Pain* can also apply to head pain, but with important exceptions that require a dedicated and more probing look. If you suffer from headaches, please refer to the Appendix for further reading. If you suffer from headaches and have not consulted anyone about them, please do.

SUMMARY:

Section III — How Do I Keep it From Happening Again?

Make Yourself Physically, Chemically and Emotionally "Fire Proof"!

"FIRE PROOF" BODY MECHANICS:

- At home
- At work
- At play

"FIRE PROOF" BODY CHEMISTRY:

Flush "Garbage" Out

- Water
- Enzymes
- Herbs

Move "Garbage" Out

- Detoxify/Eliminate
- Bodywork
- Safe Activity

Avoid "Garbage"

- pH balance
- Fatty acid balance

SUMMARY:

(Continued)

"FIRE PROOF" EMOTIONS AND MINDSET:

Stress

- Exercise
- Sleep

Outlook

- Self-image
- Worldview

CONCLUSION

What now?

NOW THAT YOU'VE COMPLETED VOLUME ONE of *Every Body's Guide to Everyday Pain*, you have at your fingertips all the information about why it hurts (Section I). You even have some ideas about how to stop it (Section II) and how to avoid it in the future (Section III). When pain comes back or a new pain shows up, as it will if you are lucky enough to see many more decades of life, just remember to stop and listen to your body. Consider the possible mechanical, chemical and emotional triggers that you learned about here.

If you've followed along and implemented as many of the ideas in this book as possible, then you've done everything that you can. It's important now to be aware that, even though you're feeling good, you're not done.

The next two volumes of this series will be key companions in your continuing efforts to remain pain free. *Volume Two: Fix the Fire Damage*, is all about how to buffer your body against all the unavoidable triggers of everyday life. It is where you'll find the strategies that will fit your situation, whether your weakness is around the mechanical, chemical or emotional stressors, or all three. *Volume Three: Plan For Fire Prevention*, is dedicated to taking the extra step and applying rehabilitation principles from Volume Two into daily life in a sustainable way.

There is no right way to do anything unless it feels right to *you*. Just because you aren't following someone else's idea of the five steps to success or the ten ways to look and feel younger or the eight days to a stress-free life doesn't mean you are doing anything wrong.

We all have our own path and we need to make peace with it. Once we do, we will find balance in our body and mind. Maybe we'll only get a glimpse of balance, but striving for it is what life is all about. Any seasoned athlete will tell you that if you fail, fall or miss the mark, you get up, dust yourself off and try it again. That's the only way to move forward, so you might as well do it armed with good information.

Despite your best efforts, you may experience the return of pain at some point in your life. You may have the same pain several times over. Hopefully you have a better understanding of what's at play. Hopefully each time you feel that pain now, you can say, "Hello old friend. You used to scare me but now I know you." Go ahead, and calmly start over. Stop, drop and roll. There's no shame in admitting to yourself that you let things slide because you felt good again for awhile. That's human nature. You have the tools. Remain calm. Be kind to yourself and just begin again.

Find "Everyday Pain Guide" on Facebook at
www.facebook.com/everydaypainguide where you can like,
follow and stay connected for the release of the next two volumes!

Beginner's Mind

"SHOSHIN" IS A JAPANESE CONCEPT POPULARLY defined by Shunryu Suzuki, a Zen master, that translates as "beginner's mind" and refers to having an attitude of openness, eagerness and lack of preconceptions when studying a subject, even when studying at an advanced level, just as a beginner in that subject would.[lxxxi] So, when you go back to the start, see if you can find that beginner's mind. Let yourself be open and eager. Above all else, make sure to be kind to yourself while you do.

Appendix

ILLUSTRATIONS

Figures

Diagrams

Photos

RESOURCES

Supporting Research

i.   Hakim AJ. Hypermobility and illness. Revised December 2013. http://hypermobility.org/help-advice/hypermobility-syndromes/what-is-hms/. Accessed December 23, 2014. *See also* Scheper MC, de Vries JE, Juul-Kristensen B, Nollet F, Engelbert RH. The functional consequences of generalized joint hypermobility: a cross-sectional study. *BMC Musculoskelet Disord.* 2014;15:243. http://www.biomedcentral.com/1471-2474/15/243. Accessed December 23, 2014.

ii.   Korting HC, Lukacs A, Vogt N, Urban J, Ehret W, Ruckdeschel G. Influence of the pH-value on the growth of Staphylococcus epidermidis, Staphylococcus aureus and Propionibacterium acnes in continuous culture. *Zentralbl Hyg Umweltmed.* 1992;93(1):78-90. *See also* Santi I, Grifantini R, Jiang SM, et al. CsrRS regulates group B *Streptococcus* virulence gene expression in response to environmental pH: a new perspective on vaccine development. *J Bacteriol.* 2009;191(17):5387-397.

iii.   Loh SH, Chen WH, Chiang CH, et al. Intracellular pH regulatory mechanism in human atrial myocardium: functional evidence for Na(+)/H(+) exchanger and Na(+)/HCO(3)(-) symporter. *J Biomed Sci.* 2002;9(3):198-205. *See also* Schwalfenberg GK. The alkaline diet: is there evidence that an

271

alkaline pH diet benefits health? *J Environ Public Health*. 2012;2012:727630. *See also* Vaughan-Jones RD, Spitzer KW, Swietach P. Intracellular pH regulation in heart. *J Mol Cell Cardiol*. 2009;46(3):318-331.

iv. Bray GE, Ying Z, Baillie LD, Zhai R, Mulligan SJ, Verge VM. Extracellular pH and neuronal depolarization serve as dynamic switches to rapidly mobilize trkA to the membrane of adult sensory neurons. *J Neurosci*. 2013;33(19):8202-8215. *See also* Ugawa S, Ueda T, Ishida Y, Nishigaki M, Shibata Y, Shimada S. Amiloride-blockable acid-sensing ion channels are leading acid sensors expressed in human nociceptors. *J Clin Invest*. 2002;110(8):1185-1190. *See also* Wu WL, Cheng CF, Sun WH, Wong CW, Chen CC. Targeting ASIC3 for pain, anxiety, and insulin resistance. *Pharmacol Ther*. 2012;134(2):127-138.

v. Birklein F, Weber M, Ernst M, Riedl B, Neundörfer B, Handwerker HO. Experimental tissue acidosis leads to increased pain in complex regional pain syndrome (CRPS). *Pain*. 2000;87(2):227-234. *See also* Lin CC, Chen WN, Chen CJ, Lin YW, Zimmer A, Chen CC. An antinociceptive role for substance P in acid-induced chronic muscle pain. *Proc Natl Acad Sci USA*. 2012;109(2):E76-E83. *See also* Steen KH, Steen AE, Kreysel HW, Reeh PW. Inflammatory mediators potentiate pain induced by experimental tissue acidosis. *Pain*. 1996;66(2-3):163-170.

vi. Gilroy DW, Colville-Nash PR, Willis D, Chivers J, Paul-Clark MJ, Willoughby DA. Inducible cyclooxygenase may have anti-inflammatory properties. *Nat Med*. 1999;5(6):698-701. *See also* Hayashi S, Ueno N, Murase A, Nakagawa Y, Takada J. Novel acid-type cyclooxygenase-2 inhibitors: design, synthesis, and structure-activity relationship for anti-inflammatory drug. *Eur J Med Chem*. 2012;50:179-195. *See also* Samad T, Abdi S. Cyclooxygenase-2 and antagonists in pain management. *Curr Opin Anaesthesiol*. 2001;14(5):527-532.

vii. Belanger L, Burt D, Callaghan J, Clifton S, Gleberzon BJ. Anterior cruciate ligament laxity related to the menstrual cycle: an updated systematic review of the literature. *J Can Chiropr Assoc*. 2013;57(1):76-86. *See also* Evans J, Salamonsen LA. Inflammation, leukocytes and menstruation. *Rev Endocr Metab Disord*. 2012;13(4):277-288. *See also* Puder JJ, Blum CA, Mueller B, De Geyter CH, Dye L, Keller U. Menstrual cycle symptoms are associated with changes in low-grade inflammation. *Eur J Clin Invest*. 2006;36(1):58-64.

viii. Bote ME, García JJ, Hinchado MD, Ortega E. Inflammatory/stress feedback dysregulation in women with fibromyalgia. *Neuroimmunomodulation*. 2012;19(6):343-351. *See also* Maes M, Kenis G, Kubera M. *Neuro Endocrinol Lett*. 2003;24(6):420-444. *See also* Ménard G, Turmel V, Bissonnette EY. Serotonin modulates the cytokine network in the lung: involvement of prostaglandin E2. *Clin Exp Immunol*. 2007;150(2):340-348.

ix. Dunlop BW, Nemeroff CB. The role of dopamine in the pathophysiology of depression. *Arch Gen Psychiatry.* 2007;64(3):327-337. *See also* Werner FM, Coveñas R. Classical neurotransmitters and neuropeptides involved in major depression in a multi-neurotransmitter system: a focus on antidepressant drugs. *Curr Med Chem.* 2013;20(38):4853-4858.

x.   Dunlop BW, Nemeroff CB. The role of dopamine in the pathophysiology of depression. *Arch Gen Psychiatry.* 2007;64(3):327-337.

xi.   Love TM. Oxytocin, motivation and the role of dopamine. *Pharmacol Biochem Behav.* 2014;119:49-60. *See also* Seligman MEP. *Learned Optimism: How to Change Your Mind and Your Life.* New York: Pocket Books; 1998. *See also* Sharot T, Shiner T, Brown AC, Fan J, Dolan RJ. Dopamine enhances expectation of pleasure in humans. *Curr Biol.* 2009;19(24):2077-2080.

xii.   Arias-Carrión O, Pöppel E. Dopamine, learning, and reward-seeking behavior. *Acta Neurobiol Exp (Wars).* 2007;67(4):481-488. *See also* Beierholm U, Guitart-Masip M, Economides M, et al. Dopamine modulates reward-related vigor. *Neuropsychopharmacology.* 2013;38(8):1495-1503. *See also* Redgrave P, Gurney K. The short-latency dopamine signal: a role in discovering novel actions? *Nat Rev Neurosci.* 2006;7(12):967-975.

xiii.   Lawrence T, Willoughby DA, Gilroy DW. Anti-inflammatory lipid mediators and insights into the resolution of inflammation. *Nat Rev Immunol.* 2002;2(10):787-795. *See also* Li CY, Chou TC, Lee CH, Tsai CS, Loh SH, Wong CS. Adrenaline inhibits lipopolysaccharide-induced macrophage inflammatory protein-1 alpha in human monocytes: the role of beta-adrenergic receptors. *Anesth Analg.* 2003;96(2):518-523.

xiv.   Karalis K, Sano H, Redwine J, Listwak S, Wilder RL, Chrousos GP. Autocrine or paracrine inflammatory actions of corticotropin-releasing hormone in vivo. *Science.* 1991;254(5030):421-423. *See also* Turnbull AV, Rivier C. Corticotropin-releasing factor, vasopressin, and prostaglandins mediate, and nitric oxide restrains, the hypothalamic-pituitary-adrenal response to acute local inflammation in the rat. *Endocrinology.* 1996;137(2):455-463.

xv.   Pert CB. *Molecules of Emotion: The Science Behind Mind-Body Medicine.* New York: Touchstone; 1999:145.

xvi.   Keleman S. *Emotional Anatomy.* Westlake Village, CA: Center Press; 1989.

xvii.   Blaurock-Busch E. Toxins and the genetic connection. *Orig Intern.* 2012;89-92. http://www.clintpublications.com/documents/September_OI_2012.pdf. Accessed December 23, 2014. *See also* Walker MR, Rapley R. Genes dictate the nature of Proteins. In: Walker MR, Rapley R. *Route Maps in Gene Technology.* Oxford, UK: Blackwell Publishing Ltd.; 2009.

xviii. Li D, Ren Y, Xu X, Zou X, Fang L, Lin Q. Sensitization of primary afferent nociceptors induced by intradermal capsaicin involves the peripheral release of calcitonin gene-related Peptide driven by dorsal root reflexes. *J Pain.* 2008;9(12):11551-1168.

xix.   Hides JA, Stokes MJ, Saide M, Jull GA, Cooper DH. Evidence of lumbar multifidus muscle wasting ipsilateral to symptoms in patients with acute/subacute low back pain. *Spine (Phila Pa 1976)*.1994;19(2):165-172.

xx. Panjabi MM. Clinical spinal instability and low back pain. *J Electromyogr Kinesiol*. 2003;13(4):371-379.

xxi. MacDonald D, Moseley GL, Hodges PW. Why do some patients keep hurting their back? Evidence of ongoing back muscle dysfunction during remission from recurrent back pain. *Pain*. 2009;142(3):183-188.

xxii. Sánchez-Zuriaga D, Adams MA, Dolan P. Is activation of the back muscles impaired by creep or muscle fatigue? *Spine (Phila Pa 1976)*. 2010;35(5):517-525.

xxiii. Purves D, Augustine GJ, Fitzpatrick D, et al. Lower motor neuron circuits and motor control. In: Purves D, Augustine GJ, Fitzpatrick D, et al, eds. *Neuroscience*. 5th ed. Sunderland, MA: Sinauer Associates, Inc.; 2012:353-374.

xxiv. Hall JE, Guyton AC. Motor functions of the spinal cord; the cord reflexes. In: Hall JE, Guyton AC. *Textbook of Medical Physiology*. 12th ed. Philadelphia, PA: Saunders Elsevier; 2011:655-666.

xxv. Cooli J. Self-treatment strategies. In: Banks C, MacKrodt. *Chronic Pain Management*. Hoboken, NJ: Wiley; 2006:221.

xxvi. Gergley JC. Acute effect of passive static stretching on lower-body strength in moderately trained men. *J Strength Cond Res*. 2013;27(4):973-977.

xxvii. Mense S. Functional anatomy of muscle: muscle, nociceptors and afferent fibers. In: Mense S, Gerwin RD, eds. *Muscle Pain: Understanding the Mechanisms*. New York: Springer-Verlag; 2010:17-48.

xxviii. Kingston B. *Understanding Joints: A Practical Guide to Their Structure and Function*. Cheltenham: Stanley Thornes; 2000. *See also* Matsen FA III, ed; University of Washington. Joints. Updated 2011. http://www.orthop.washington.edu/?q=patient-care/articles/arthritis/joints.html. Accessed December 23, 2013.

xxix. Mann EM, Carr EC. *Pain: Creative Approaches to Effective Management*. 2nd ed. New York: Palgrave Macmillan; 2009.

xxx. Knobloch K, Grasemann R, Spies M, Vogt PM. Intermittent KoldBlue cryotherapy of 3x10 min changes mid-portion Achilles tendon microcirculation. *Br J Sports Med*. 2007;41(6):e4.

xxxi. Martin M. Chill out: warmth may be more inviting, but cooling might be just what that injury needs. *Pacific Northwest Magazine*. Published 2002. http://seattletimes.com/pacificnw/2002/0609/fitness.html. Accessed December 23, 2014.

xxxii. Ogura T, Tashiro M, Masud M, Watanuki S, Shibuya K, Yamaguchi K, et al. Cerebral metabolic changes in men after chiropractic spinal manipulation for neck pain. *Altern Ther Health Med*. 2011;17(6):12-17.

xxxiii. Zijlstra FJ1, van den Berg-de Lange I, Huygen FJ, Klein J. Anti-inflammatory actions of acupuncture. *Mediators Inflamm*. 2003;12(2):59-69.

xxxiv. Simpson N, Dinges DF. Sleep and inflammation. *Nutr Rev.* 2007;65(12 pt 2): S244-S252.

xxxv. Srivastava KC, Mustafa T. Ginger (Zingiber officinale) in rheumatism and musculoskeletal disorders. *Med Hypoth.* 1992;39(4):342-348. *See also* Arora RB, Basu N, Kapoor V, et al. Anti-inflammatory studies on Curcuma longa (turmeric). *Indian J Med Res.* 1971;59(8):1289-1295.

xxxvi. Ammon HP, Safayhi H, Mack T, Sabieraj J. Mechanism of antiinflammatory actions of curcumine and boswellic acids. *J Ethnopharmacol* 1993;38(2-3): 113-119.

xxxvii. Harvard Medical School. What you eat can fuel or cool inflammation, a key driver of heart disease, diabetes, and other chronic conditions. Updated February 2007. http://www.health.harvard.edu/fhg/updates/What-you-eat-can-fuel-or-cool-inflammation-a-key-driver-of-heart-disease-diabetes-and-other-chronic-conditions.shtml. Accessed December 23, 2014. *See also* Bauer B. Buzzed on inflammation. *Mayo Clin Hlth Lett.* http://healthletter. mayoclinic.com/editorial/editorial.cfm/i/163/t/Buzzed%20on%20 inflammation/. Accessed December 23, 2014.

xxxviii. Lopez-Garcia E, van Dam RM, Qi L, Hu FB. Coffee consumption and markers of inflammation and endothelial dysfunction in healthy and diabetic women. *Am J Clin Nutr.* 2006;84(4):888-893.

xxxix. Simpson N, Dinges DF. Sleep and inflammation. *Nutr Rev.* 2007;65(12 pt 2): S244-S252.

xl. Baessler A, Nadeem R, Harvey M, Madbouly E, Younus A, Sajid H, et al. Treatment for sleep apnea by continuous positive airway pressure improves levels of inflammatory markers - a meta analysis. *J Inflamm (Lond.).* 2013;10:13.

xli. Hauser RA. The acceleration of articular cartilage degeneration in osteoarthritis by nonsteroidal anti-inflammatory drugs. *J Prolother.* 2010;2(1):305-322. http://www.journalofprolotherapy.com/index.php/ the-acceleration-of-articular-cartilage-degeneration-in-osteoarthritis-by-nonsteroidal-anti-inflammatory-drugs/. Accessed December 23, 2014.

xlii. Linton AL. Adverse effects of NSAIDs on renal function. *Can Med Assoc J.* 1984;131(3):189-191. *See also* Musu M, Finco G, Antonucci R, Polati E, Sanna D, Evangelista M, et al. Acute nephrotoxicity of NSAID from the foetus to the adult. *Eur Rev Med Pharmacol Sci.* 2011;15(12):1461-1472. *See also* Simon LS. Nonsteroidal anti-inflammatory drugs and their risk: a story still in development. *Arthritis Res Ther.* 2013;15(suppl 3):S1.

xliii. US National Library of Medicine. LiverTox: clinical and research information on drug-induced liver injury. Drug record: nonsteroidal antiinflammatory drugs. Updated November 11, 2014. http://livertox.nih. gov/NonsteroidalAntiinflammatoryDrugs.htm. Accessed December 23, 2014. *See also* Lewis JH. Hepatic toxicity of nonsteroidal anti-inflammatory drugs. *Clin Pharm.* 1984;3(2):128-138. *See also* Bessone F. Non-steroidal anti-inflammatory drugs: What is the actual risk of liver damage? *World J Gastroenterol.* 2010;16(45):5651-5661.

xliv. Mellemkjaer L, Blot WJ, Sørensen HT, Thomassen L, McLaughlin JK, Nielsen GL, et al. Upper gastrointestinal bleeding among users of NSAIDs: a population-based cohort study in Denmark. *Br J Clin Pharmacol.* 2002;53(2):173-181.

xlv. van den Bemt P, Tjwa ET, van Oijen MG. Cardiovascular and gastrointestinal safety of NSAIDs. [In Dutch]. *Ned Tijdschr Geneeskd.* 2014;158:A7311. *See also* Singh BK, Haque SE, Pillai KK. Assessment of nonsteroidal anti-inflammatory drug-induced cardiotoxicity. *Expert Opin Drug Metab Toxicol.* 2014;10(2):143-156.

xlvi. Malliaropoulos N, Isinkaye T, Tsitas K, Maffulli N. Reinjury after acute posterior thigh muscle injuries in elite track and field athletes [Erratum in *Am J Sports Med.* 2011;39(4):NP7]. *Am J Sports Med.* 2011;39(2):304-310.

xlvii. American Academy of Orthopaedic Surgeons. Effects of aging. Updated September 2009. http://orthoinfo.aaos.org/topic.cfm?topic=A00191. Accessed December 23, 2014. *See also* Besdine RW, ed. Changes in the body with aging. In: *Merck Manual.* Whitehouse Station, NJ: Merck Sharp & Dohme Corp.; 2013. http://www.merckmanuals.com/home/older_peoples_health_issues/the_aging_body/changes_in_the_body_with_aging.html. Accesed December 23, 2014.

xlviii. Tskhovrebova L, Trinick J. Roles of titin in the structure and elasticity of the sarcomere. *J Biomed Biotechnol.* 2010;2010:612482.

xlix. Linke WA, Krüger M. The giant protein titin as an integrator of myocyte signaling pathways. *Physiology (Bethesda).* 2010;25(3):186-198.

l. Bellafiore M, Cappello F, Palumbo D, Macaluso F, Bianco A, Palma A, et al. Increased expression of titin in mouse gastrocnemius muscle in response to an endurance-training program. *Eur J Histochem.* 2007;51(2):119-124.

li. Antczak A, Ciebiada M, Kharitonov SA, Gorski P, Barnes PJ. Inflammatory markers: exhaled nitric oxide and carbon monoxide during the ovarian cycle. *Inflammation.* 2012;35(2):554-559.

lii. Tait AS, Butts CL, Sternberg EM. The role of glucocorticoids and progestins in inflammatory, autoimmune, and infectious disease *J Leukoc Biol.* 2008;84(4):924-931.

liii. Puder JJ, Blum CA, Mueller B, De Geyter Ch, Dye L, et al. Menstrual cycle symptoms are associated with changes in low-grade inflammation. *Eur J Clin Invest.* 2006;36(1):58-64.

liv. Imam TH, ed. Overview of urinary tract infections. In: *Merck Manual.* http://www.merckmanuals.com/home/kidney_and_urinary_tract_disorders/urinary_tract_infections_uti/overview_of_urinary_tract_infections.html. Whitehouse Station, NJ: Merck Sharp & Dohm Corp; 2014. Accessed

December 23, 2014. *See also* Grabe M, Bishop MC, Bjerklund-Johansen, Botto H, Cek M, Lobel B, et al; European Association of Urology. *Guidelines on the Management of Urinary and Male Genital Tract Infections.* 2008. http://www.uroweb.org/fileadmin/user_upload/Guidelines/The%20 Management%20of%20Male%20Urinary%20and%20Genital%20Tract%20 Infections.pdf. Accessed December 23, 2014.

lv. Gaskins AJ, Wilchesky M, Mumford SL, Whitcomb BW, Browne RW, Wactawski-Wende J, et al. Endogenous reproductive hormones and C-reactive protein across the menstrual cycle: the BioCycle study. *Am J Epidemiol.* 2012;175(5):423-431.

lvi. Drake VJ; Oregon State University. Nutrition and inflammation. Published 2010. http://lpi.oregonstate.edu/infocenter/inflammation.html. Accessed December 23, 2014. *See also* Bauer B. Buzzed on inflammation. *Mayo Clin Hlth Lett.* http://healthletter.mayoclinic.com/editorial/editorial.cfm/i/163/t/ Buzzed%20on%20inflammation/. Accessed December 23, 2014.

lvii. Calder PC. Omega-3 polyunsaturated fatty acids and inflammatory processes: nutrition or pharmacology? *Br J Clin Pharmacol.* 2013;75(3):645-662.

lviii. Tursi JM, Phair PG, Barnes GL. Plant sources of acid stable lipases: potential therapy for cystic fibrosis [Erratum in *J Paediatr Child Health.* 1995;31(4):364]. *J Paediatr Child Health.* 1994;30(6):539-543.

lix. Saller R, Iten F, Reichling J. Dyspeptic pain and phytotherapy--a review of traditional and modern herbal drugs [In German]. *Forsch Komplementarmed Klass Naturheilkd.* 2001;8(5):263-273.

lx. Calder PC. The role of marine omega-3 (n-3) fatty acids in inflammatory processes, atherosclerosis and plaque stability. *Mol Nutr Food Res.* 2012;56(7):1073-1080.

lxi. Welty FK. How do elevated triglycerides and low HDL-cholesterol affect inflammation and atherothrombosis? *Curr Cardiol Rep.* 2013;15(9):400.

lxii. Simopoulos AP. The importance of the ratio of omega-6/omega-3 essential fatty acids. *Biomed Pharmacother.* 2002;56(8):365-79.

lxiii. Simopoulos AP. The importance of the ratio of omega-6/omega-3 essential fatty acids. *Biomed Pharmacother.* 2002;56(8):365-79.

lxiv. Castro-González MI, Méndez-Armenta M. Heavy metals: Implications associated to fish consumption. *Environ Toxicol Pharmacol.* 2008;26(3): 263-271.

lxv. Owen C. *An Endocrine Interpretation of Chapman's Reflexes.* Indianapolis, IN: American Academy of Osteopathy; 1937. *See also* Capobianco JD. In: DiGiovanna EL, Schiowitz S, Dowling DJ, eds. *An Osteopathic Approach to Diagnosis and Treatment.* 3rd ed. Philadelphia, PA: Lippincott Williams and Wilkins; 2005.

lxvi. Quach CJ. Relationship between Chapman's reflexes and acupuncture meridians by traditional Chinese medicine practitioners in Taiwan. http://www.

osteopathic.org/inside-aoa/development/international-osteopathic-medicine/ Documents/Relationship%20Between%20Chapman%27s%20Reflexes%20 and%20Acupuncture%20Meridians%20by%20Traditional%20Chinese%20 Medicine%20Practitioners%20in%20Taiwan.pdf. Accessed December 23, 2014. *See also* Stone CA. Visceral and Obstetric Osteopathy. Philadelphia, PA: Elsevier; 2007:52-53. *See also* Chila A. *Foundations of Osteopathic Medicine.* Philadelphia, PA: Lippincott Williams & Wilkins; 2010.

lxvii.   Beinfield B, Korngold E. *Between Heaven and Earth: A Guide to Chinese Medicine.* New York: Random House Publishing; 1991:67-70.

lxviii.   Leknes SG, Bantick S, Willis CM, Wilkinson JD, Wise RG, Tracey I. Itch and motivation to scratch: an investigation of the central and peripheral correlates of allergen- and histamine-induced itch in humans. *J Neurophysiol.* 2007;97(1):415-422.

lxix.   Anxiety and Depression Society of America. Physical activity reduces stress. http://www.adaa.org/understanding-anxiety/related-illnesses/other-related-conditions/stress/physical-activity-reduces-st. Accessed December 23, 2014. *See also* National Center for Complementary and Alternative Medicine. Relaxation techniques for health: an introduction. http://nccam.nih.gov/ health/stress/relaxation.htm. Accessed December 23, 2014.

lxx.   Shapiro F. *Eye Movement Desensitization and Reprocessing: Basic Principles, Protocols and Procedures.* 1st ed. New York: Guilford Press; 1995.

lxxi.   Schoenfeld TJ, Rada P, Pieruzzini PR, Hsueh B, Gould E. Physical exercise prevents stress-induced activation of granule neurons and enhances local inhibitory mechanisms in the dentate gyrus. *J Neurosci.* 2013;33(18): 7770-7777.

lxxii.   Seligman ME, Czikszentmihalyi M. Positive psychology. An introduction. *Am Psychol.* 2000;55(1):5-14.

lxxiii.   Csikszentmihalyi M. Finding Flow: The Psychology of Engagement with Everyday Life. New York: HarperCollins Publishers, Inc.; 1997.

lxxiv.   Lockly SW, Foster RG. *Sleep. A Very Short Introduction.* New York: Oxford University Press; 2012. *See also* Alfarra R, Fins AI, Chayo I, Tartar JL. Changes in attention to an emotional task after sleep deprivation: Neurophysiological and behavioral findings. *Biol Psychol.* 2014;104C:1-7. *See also* Liu JC, Verhulst S, Massar SA, Chee MW. Sleep deprived and sweating it out: the effects of total sleep deprivation on skin conductance reactivity to psychosocial stress. *Sleep.* 2015; 38(1):155-159.

lxxv.   Neckelmann D, Mykletun A, Dahl AA. Chronic insomnia as a risk factor for developing anxiety and depression. *Sleep.* 2007;30(7):873-880.

lxxvi.   Mullington JM, Simpson NS, Meier-Ewert HK, Haack M. Sleep loss and inflammation. *Best Pract Res Clin Endocrinol Metab.* 2010;24(5):775-784.

lxxvii.   Lockly SW, Foster RG. *Sleep. A Very Short Introduction.* New York: Oxford University Press; 2012.

lxxviii. Mednick SC, Cai DJ, Kanady J, Drummond SP. Comparing the benefits of caffeine, naps and placebo on verbal, motor and perceptual memory. *Behav Brain Res.* 2008;193(1):79-86.

lxxix. Reavley NJ, Pilkington PD. Use of Twitter to monitor attitudes toward depression and schizophrenia: an exploratory study. *PeerJ.* 2014;2:e647. *See also* Barry CL, McGinty EE. Stigma and public support for parity and government spending on mental health: a 2013 national opinion survey. *Psychiatr Serv.* 2014;65(10):1265-1268.

lxxx. British Association for Counselling & Psychotherapy. Increase in counselling and psychotherapy suggests lessening of mental health stigma. Published July 7, 2014. http://www.bacp.co.uk/media/?newsId=3506. Accessed December 23, 2014. *See also* Segal SP, Silverman C, Temkin T. Empowerment and self-help agency practice for people with mental disabilities. *Soc Work.* 1993;38(6):705-12.

lxxxi. Suzuki S. *Zen Mind, Beginner's Mind.* Tokyo: John Weatherhill; 1970.

RESOURCES

Recommended Reading

For More on the Mechanics of Everyday Pain

Edwards MZ. *YogAlign, Pain-Free Yoga From Your Inner Core.* Hanalei, HI: Hihimanu Press; 2011.

Gokhale E, Adams S. *8 Steps to a Pain-Free Back: Natural Posture Solutions for Pain in the Back, Neck, Shoulder, Hip, Knee, and Foot.* Chicago, IL: Pendo Press; 2008.

Hage M. *The Back Pain Book.* Pompano Beach, FL: Educa Books; 2008.

Liebenson C. *Flexibility, Yoga Training, and Ergonomic Postural Advice.* Published on DVD. Riverwoods, IL: Wolters Kluwer Heath; 2011.

McGill S. *Back Mechanic: The Step-by-Step McGill Method to Fix Back Pain.* Waterloo, Ontario: Stuart McGill Wabuno Publishers; 2015.

McGill S. *Ultimate Back Fitness and Performance.* 5th ed. Waterloo, Ontario: Stuart McGill Wabuno Publishers; 2004.

McKenzie RA. *Treat Your Own Back.* 9th ed. Orthopedic Physical Therapy Products Orthopedic Physical Therapy Products; 2011.

Myers T. Anatomy Trains website. https://www.anatomytrains.com.

Roland M, Waddel G, Moffett JK, Burton K, Main C. *The Back Book: The Best Way to Deal With Back Pain.* Norwich, UK: The Stationary Office; 2002.(http://www.newtonplacesurgery.nhs.uk/website/G82039/files/BackBookEnglish.pdf)

Schleip R, ed. *Fascia: The Tensional Network of the Human Body.* New York: Churchill Livingston/Elsevier; 2012.

Snell P. Fix Your Own Back website. http://www.fixyourownback.com.

For More on the Chemistry and Biology of Everyday Pain

Abascal K. To Quiet Inflammation website. http://toquietinflammation.com.

Alschuler L, Gazella KA. *The Definitive Guide to Thriving After Cancer.* Revised ed. Berkeley, CA: Ten Speed Press; 2013.

Baillie-Hamilton P. Toxic Overload: *A Doctor's Plan for Combating the Illnesses Caused by Chemicals in Our Foods, Our Homes, and Our Medicine Cabinets.* New York: Avery; 2005.

Bland J. *The Disease Delusion: Conquering Causes of Chronic Illness for a Healthier, Longer, and Happier Life.* New York: HarperWave; 2014.

Blaylock RL. *Health and Nutrition Secrets that Can Save Your Life.* Albuquerque, NM: Health Press; 2006.

Buchholz M. *Heal Your Headache: The 1-2-3 Program for Taking Charge of Your Pain.* New York: Workman Publishing; 2002.

Dowd J. *The Vitamin D Cure*. Hoboken, NJ: John Wiley & Sons; 2012.

Enders G, Enders J. *Gut: The Inside Story of Our Body's Most Underrated Organ*. Vancouver: Greystone Books; 2015.

Gutman J. *Glutathione Your Key to Health*. Canada: Kudo.ca Communications; 2008.

Holick. *The Vitamin D Solution: A 3-Step Strategy to Cure Our Most Common Health Problem*. New York: Hudson Street Press; 2010.

Hyman M. *The Blood Sugar Solution: The Ultrahealthy Program for Losing Weight, Preventing Disease, and Feeling Great Now*. Emmaus PA: Rodale; 2012.

Moseley L. *Painful Yarns: Metaphors & Stories to Help Understand the Biology of Pain*. Minneapolis, MN: Orthopedic Physical Therapy Products; 2007.

Murray MT, Pizzorno JE. *The Encyclopedia of Natural Medicine*. New York: Atria Books; 2012.

Murray MT, Pizzorno JE, Pizzorno L. *The Encyclopedia of Healing Foods*. New York: Avery; 2005.

Naidu AS. *Redox Life*. Pomona, CA: Bio-Rep Media; 2013.

O'Connell J. *Sugar Nation: The Hidden Truth Behind America's Deadliest Habit and the Simple Way to Beat It*. New York: Hyperion; 2010.

Perlmutter D, Colman C. *The Better Brain Book*. London: Penguin Books; 2005.

Pollan M. *In Defense of Food: An Eater's Manifesto*. London: Penguin Books; 2008.

Sears B. *The Anti-Inflammation Zone: Reversing the Silent Epidemic That's Destroying Our Health*. New York: ReganBooks; 2005.

Sisson M. *The Primal Blueprint*. Malibu, CA: Primal Blueprint Publishing; 2013.

Wahls TL, Adamson E. *The Wahls Protocol: How I Beat Progressive MS Using Paleo Principles and Functional Medicine*. New York: Avery; 2014.

Weil A. *Healthy Aging: A Lifelong Guide to Your Well-Being*. Mississauga, Ontario: Random House of Canada; 2005.

Yasko A. *Genetic Bypass: Using Nutrition to Bypass Genetic Mutations*. United States: Matrix Development Publishing; 2005.

For More on the Emotions of Everyday Pain

Borysenko J. *Minding the Body, Mending the Mind*. New York: MJF Books; 2014.

Keleman S. *Emotional Anatomy*. Westlake Village, CA: Center Press; 1989.

Lipton BH. *The Biology of Belief: Unleashing the Power of Consciousness, Matter & Miracles*. Carlsbad, CA: Hay House; 2015.

Myss MC. *Why People Don't Heal and How They Can*. New York: Harmony Books; 1997.

Pert CB. *Molecules of Emotion: Why You Feel the Way You Feel*. New York: Scribner; 1997.

Sapolsky RM. *Why Zebras Don't Get Ulcers*. 3rd ed. New York: Times Books; 2014.

Sarno JE. *Healing Back Pain: The Mind-Body Connection*. New York: Warner Books; 1991.

Selye H. *The Stress of Life: A Scientist's Memoirs*. 2nd ed. New York: Van Nostrand Reinhold; 1979.

Sternberg EM. *The Balance Within: The Science Connecting Health and Emotions*. New York: Freeman; 2000.

INDEX

Page numbers with an *n* denote a footnote.

ACKNOWLEDGMENTS

Reflections of Gratitude

ASIDE FROM THE DECADES SPENT INCUBATING these ideas and gathering life experience while enjoying peaceful private practice, the written and illustrated aspect of this project has been the better part of five years in the making. During this time I've had the good fortune of stumbling upon the remarkable talents of several kind and generous women who also call the Pacific Northwest home. I take pleasure in fostering work relationships local to the part of the world that happens to make my heart sing.

There simply would be no book without the very early encouragement by **Nancy Wick** who gave me the kind and subtle nudges I needed to spark my vision. It wasn't until after she looked over a very rough outline and early chapter draft that I felt any inkling this book could have the bones necessary to become reality rather than just a stapled, collated paper handout. Thanks also to my early readers, Mary and Karen, who, despite their very full lives, were willing to give me valuable casual feedback.

Sandy Johnson is the extraordinary magician of an illustrator responsible for bringing my words to life with her uncanny creative sense. She somehow knew from the start exactly what I was trying to convey visually. Unflinchingly, she proceeded to digest and promptly translate volumes of my thoughts and imaginations in words into replicas of my vision. The playful nuances captured by her images seem to flow directly from my own mind, which is habitually filled with light-hearted animated analogies of everyday things. I couldn't have hoped for a more seamless process. Her images continue to make me smile even on the umpteenth reread and review.

Sherri Damlo's watchful eye is to thank not only for the final sweep of this manuscript in its entirety but in particular for assuring that my claims have basis in studied fact as much as was possible. Throughout the years I've had to do my share of dabbling in the art of deciphering scientific literature, but it's out of necessity more than with any of the formal studied skill of someone who makes a living at research editing. Sherri gets my utmost respect for making her work seem easy, which it most certainly is not.

Ultimately, the experience of teaching has been the formative influence behind this book series. Teaching both massage students and student doctors of naturopathy, is what forced me to learn how to distill what in academia are widely compartmentalized and complex ideas about anatomy, physiology, kinesiology and physical medicine. What I came to appreciate in the process is how much the true understanding of our own body lies in the ability to view those compartments as a whole, which is the only way to grasp the impact they have on each other—in and out of balance. We are the sum of our compartments and no one knows that better than the Bastyr University graduates who had the great misfortune (tongue in cheek) of class time with me in the physical medicine department. To them I owe thanks for their influence in shaping the goal for all three volumes of *Every Body's Guide to Everyday Pain*. The student doctors at Bastyr helped me appreciate where I also once was in the learning process—at which point compartmental thinking is essential for learning and yet brilliantly distorts the big picture. That insightful "wholeistic," big picture for me only came into full focus after meaningful time spent in clinical practice combined with the experience of teaching. Both my students and patients have taught me about where we *all* are in the process of getting to know our own body, and where each of us—doctors and patients alike—have the potential to be with our own command of this information once it's properly decoded.

The very beginning of my own path in the clinical setting outside of school began in Connecticut at the gracious doorstep of my first chiropractic employer **Sharon Vallone, DC**. She saw in me potential that I could not have realized on my own nor without the incredible leap of faith she took in hiring me. She entrusted the care of her dear patients to me—a complete stranger fresh out of school. What I learned working in her practice fundamentally influences and shapes my style of practice to this very day. Not a day goes by that I don't think of each and every one of the Tolland and Hartford Westside Chiropractic clan who worked alongside me in that office and helped me succeed and grow.

Finally I cannot forget to express my affection and admiration for the two sweet young women who helped to fill the pages of my books with the photographic material integral for the core of what this project needs in order to communicate and guide readers through the pain-troubleshooting process. I'm impatient and excited to show more of their work in Volumes Two and Three. Thank you to **Hayden Fidler** and **Chelsea Grace** for your cheerful ease and sweet spirits!

SPECIAL THANKS

THESE ARE THE PEOPLE WHO LIFTED me up in unexpected ways at the eleventh hour. They all went out of their way to help this project become a reality.

Your kindness will not be forgotten:

- Erica Wolf Esq.
- Victoria Colotta
- James T. Egan
- Cathy Lewis

Also a special thank you to Bob Majors, Nadine Waldmann, Shannon Flynn, Paula Fedirchuk, Emily Fowler, Susan Turner, Tiffany Clark, Kristi Jordan, Victoria Scott, Jen Jarta, Erica Sternin, Babara Parnell, Arlene Strong, Heidi Edwards, Mihal Ehven, Ellen Garduno, Dina Tanners, Tina Ilvonen, Diana Thompson, Michelle Briscoe, Heidi Page, Frankie Marazzi, Alex L. Alexander, Emi Mizuki, Chiyo Ishikawa, Judith Leconte, Jane D. Saxton, and Jerri Ninesling. You all took the time to read/review the book for me, and for that, I am truly grateful.

ABOUT THE AUTHOR

YA-LING J. LIOU, DC, is a chiropractic physician who, after more than 20 years of clinical experience, continues to expand and share her intuitive body care techniques. All of her work takes into account the whole person, aiming not only to address the mechanical balance of the body, but also the chemical and emotional aspects that so often influence this balance.

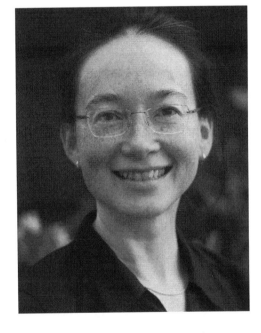

Growing up with exposure to generations of Eastern as well as Western attitudes toward health provided Dr. Liou with a unique perspective on health care. She began her formal education in the area of applied sciences in her hometown of Montreal, Quebec, before completing a degree program at New York Chiropractic College.

Dr. Liou now lives, works and writes in Seattle. She taught anatomy, physiology and kinesiology at Seattle Massage School (currently Everest College and formerly Ashmead College), and later brought her multiple systems perspective to the Naturopathic Physical Medicine Department at Bastyr University as an adjunct faculty member.

STAY CONNECTED!

Want to find out more about the author?
Join her online today!

🏠 www.returntohealth.org

me https://about.me/drliou

🐦 @yalingliou

f www.facebook.com/yaling.lioudc

in https://www.linkedin.com/in/yalingliou

✉ http://eepurl.com/bCy_Rr

Looking for more about *Everyday Pain Guide* and the next two volumes? Visit the official Facebook Page at www.facebook.com/everydaypainguide.